BEYOND FLEXNER

Recent Titles in
Contributions in Medical Studies

Beyond Flexner

MEDICAL EDUCATION IN THE TWENTIETH CENTURY

EDITED BY
Barbara Barzansky
AND
Norman Gevitz

Contributions in Medical Studies, Number 34

GREENWOOD PRESS
New York • Westport, Connecticut • London

Library of Congress Cataloging-in-Publication Data

Beyond Flexner : medical education in the twentieth century / edited
  by Barbara Barzansky and Norman Gevitz.
      p.   cm.—(Contributions in medical studies, ISSN 0886–8220 ;
  no. 34)
    "Outgrowth of a conference held at the University of Illinois
College of Medicine in June 1986." —Pref.
    Includes bibliographical references and index.
    ISBN 0–313–25984–4 (alk. paper)
    1. Medical education—United States—History—Congresses.
2. Flexner, Abraham, 1866–1959. Medical education in the United
States and Canada—Congresses. I. Barzansky, Barbara M.
II. Gevitz, Norman. III. University of Illinois at Chicago.
College of Medicine. IV. Series.
R745.B46   1992
610'.71'173—dc20   91–24333

British Library Cataloguing in Publication Data is available.

Library of Congress Catalog Card Number: 91–24333
ISBN: 0–313–25984–4
ISSN: 0886–8220

First published in 1992

Greenwood Press, 88 Post Road West, Westport, CT 06881
An imprint of Greenwood Publishing Group, Inc.

Printed in the United States of America

∞™

The paper used in this book complies with the
Permanent Paper Standard issued by the National
Information Standards Organization (Z39.48–1984).

10 9 8 7 6 5 4 3 2 1

Copyright Acknowledgments

The chapter by Mary Roth Walsh was published in the July 1990 issue of
the *New York State Journal of Medicine* 90 (6): 302–6. Permission to include
this material is gratefully acknowledged.

Contents

Illustrations

Acknowledgments

This book is an outgrowth of a conference held at the University of Illinois College of Medicine in June 1986, commemorating the seventy-fifth anniversary of publication of the "Flexner Report," *Medical Education in the United States and Canada*. The editors wish to thank Ronald Richards, Ph.D., then director of the Center for Educational Development of the University of Illinois at Chicago and currently of the W. K. Kellogg Foundation, for his support and encouragement. Sincere appreciation is also extended to Phillip Forman, M.D., then dean of the University of Illinois College of Medicine, for providing financial support for the conference and to Carlos J. M. Martini, M.D., M.P.H., vice president for medical education at the American Medical Association, who arranged AMA funding for and co-sponsorship of this event.

Introduction

For decades, educators, historians, and social commentators accorded to the "Flexner Report" major responsibility for the reform of the medical education system in the United States. In recent years, however, a number of historians have both challenged the impact of the report and questioned the desirability of the changes in medical education that were attributed to it. Some of the revisionist arguments are grounded in new research about the educational reforms at leading schools in the half-century prior to Flexner's study and the activities of organizations such as the American Medical Association, the Association of American Medical Colleges, and the Federation of State Medical Boards around the time of the report. In contrast, the distinguished scholar Thomas Bonner has forcefully argued that many historians in the 1970s and 1980s with "a strong presentist perspective" have fashioned their positions on ideology rather than new knowledge, and thus have blamed Flexner for a variety of problems in modern medical education. According to Bonner, such revisionist writing has been characterized by "an extravagance of language, a political partisanship, and a shrillness of tone unknown a generation before." Whether or not one agrees with Bonner's assessment, an undeniable point is that among historians and medical educators the Flexner Report still generates much heated debate.

The goal of this volume is to trace a number of elements articulated in the "Flexner Report" as they evolved during the twentieth century. Flexner's ideas on medical education serve as a "lens" through which one can observe and evaluate the many changes that have occurred in the past eighty years. While the recent important works by Kenneth Ludmerer, *Learning to Heal* (New York: Basic Books, 1985) and William Rothstein, *American Medical Schools and the Practice of Medicine* (New York: Oxford University Press, 1987) have extended our knowledge of the structure and process of medical education, they do not exhaust the subject, nor do they deal in depth with a number of significant topics examined by contributors to this book.

In his introductory essay, Robert P. Hudson establishes the social context of the "Flexner Report," describing the changes that were already underway in American medical education and the forces that were influencing its development. He considers Flexner's goals for reform and his catalytic effect in shaping the current form of medical education. In addition, Hudson examines the myths that have arisen in conjunction with the "Flexner Report," discusses the arguments of critics who have offered radical interpretations of the meaning of reform, and provides his own evaluation of Flexner's contributions.

In examining the development of medical education in the twentieth century, comparatively little attention has been directed at the basic science years. In her chapter, "The Growth and Divergence of the Basic Sciences," Barbara Barzansky examines the state of the preclinical curriculum at the time of the "Flexner Report" and at fifteen-year intervals to the present. She describes the amount of time devoted to the various basic sciences and the proportion of time in each discipline devoted to laboratory teaching. Barzansky focuses on several themes, including the controversies over the applied versus discipline-based orientation of the basic sciences and the proper training of preclinical faculty members. She also traces opinions about curricular problems and describes the solutions that were proposed by leaders in medical education.

Edward C. Atwater's essay on clinical education since Flexner is subtitled "Whatever Became of William Osler?" Atwater identifies four major changes that have affected clinical teaching in this century: the establishment of university control over hospitals, with the subsequent replacement of the practitioner by the full-time subspecialist as a role model for students; the expansion of sophisticated technology and biomedical knowledge, which promoted specialism; the passing of financial control from individuals and philanthropies to third parties; and the increased willingness of the public to spend money on health. Atwater looks at the effects of these elements, which he notes have not always been salutary, on the sites used for teaching, the clinical curriculum, the patients, the teachers, and the students.

In her chapter, "Women in Medicine Since Flexner," Mary Roth Walsh challenges the position of some historians that the "Flexner Report" was a major explanation for the subsequent decrease in the number of women physicians. She documents the structural and psychological barriers established in the nineteenth century against women becoming medical students and notes that women welcomed the efforts of the reform movement to raise standards. However, the merging and closing of women's medical colleges resulted in a decline in the total number of women graduates, since medical schools that opened their doors to women adopted a deliberate policy to exclude all but a few. Finally, Walsh looks at the reasons for the recent increase in the number of women in medical school and considers still unresolved issues of discrimination on the basis of gender.

While the number of black medical schools declined from ten to seven in the period between 1900 and 1910, Todd L. Savitt notes that the appearance of the "Flexner Report" directly affected the fate of the remaining institutions. Black medical schools came to be subject to the higher standards and requirements mandated by the American Medical Association's Council on Medical Education and the state medical boards, yet they were initially denied the aid necessary to upgrade themselves. Philanthropies, including the General Education Board, placed priorities on funding elite white schools. As the black colleges hovered between life and death, the Council on Medical Education and the General Education Board argued over who should take the first step to save the two strongest institutions—Howard and Meharry. Though Flexner was eventually instrumental in obtaining funding for both schools, the demise of the other black colleges reduced the number of black physicians at a time when the need for such practitioners was increasing.

While black schools were dramatically affected by the "Flexner Report" and the activities of the Council on Medical Education, osteopathic schools, also included in the Flexner survey, were not. Norman Gevitz, in "The Fate of Sectarian Medical Education," argues that osteopathic colleges provide a comparative example through which the forces for change in medical education can better be appreciated. He notes that homeopathic and eclectic medical schools, which had been in trouble prior to 1910, ultimately failed because they could not maintain autonomy over their educational standards, could not achieve economic solvency, and could not attract sufficient numbers of students. The number of osteopathic schools only declined from eight to seven in the 25 years after the Flexner Report, because the American Osteopathic Association (AOA) did not enforce a rapid pace of reform. It was only due to external pressures, particularly the threat in some states of the loss of AOA accrediting power combined with the desire of practitioners for an expanded scope of practice, that osteopathic schools began to reform.

Medical education is not a closed system. It should be dependent upon and reflective of the nature of the health care delivery system. In his chapter, "American Health Services Since the Flexner Report," Odin W. Anderson provides an overview of the fundamental changes that have taken place over the past century. He identifies three periods. The first (1875–1930) involved the development of the infrastructure, when the voluntary hospital movement flourished. This was followed by the era of third party reimbursement, which saw the emergence of private health insurance plans and the implementation of Medicare and Medicaid in the mid–1960s. We presently are, and will continue to be, in the era of management and control. The question now being posed is how can health care costs be reduced without sacrificing quality of care. As Anderson notes, the strategies for cost control that have been adopted or are being considered bear on the content and direction of medical education.

As Janet D. Perloff notes in "Trends in the Financing of Undergraduate Medical Education," by the late 1950s federal research grants and contracts accounted for 25 percent of medical school revenues. As a result, the number of full-time faculty members increased, and these individuals devoted the majority of their time to research rather than to teaching. In the 1960s, new sources of federal funding were provided to meet the perceived physician shortage. These funding programs fostered curriculum and faculty development, specifically the expansion of programs to train primary care providers. By 1980, perceptions of physician oversupply were common and the sources of funding to increase manpower had mostly disappeared. The past two decades have seen the expansion of faculty practice plans, which are playing an increasing role in financing medical education. Perloff examines the consequences of this recent shift in funding, and considers proposals to deal with the potential negative impact on education.

Barbara Barzansky and Janet D. Perloff next consider "Trends in the Use of Outpatient Settings for Medical Education." They note that during the Flexner period outpatient settings were widely used, but many believed that the care provided and the opportunities for student learning were inferior to those on the hospital ward. Outpatient physicians usually were junior faculty members, with lower status and little contact with their peers on inpatient services. Barzansky and Perloff describe a number of models of outpatient teaching that have been tried: the preceptorship, the comprehensive clinic, and the health maintenance organization. The benefits of these sites, and the problems identified with their use, are discussed.

In his chapter, "The Medical Curriculum: Developments and Directions," DeWitt C. Baldwin, Jr. identifies three sources of educational innovation: the profession itself, the social and economic environment, and the structure and content of medicine. Specifically, he examines the roles of the American Medical Association and the Association of American Medical Colleges, state and federal legislation, changing patterns of health services and the new practice environment, the growth of specialties, and the development of new knowledge and technology. He describes the increasing length and content of the curriculum, changes in philosophy and experimental methods of teaching, the development of alternate curricular tracks, and the appearance of new subject areas.

Finally, he considers whether recent alterations in the curriculum are likely to result in graduates able to meet society's needs.

Given the dynamic relationship between our training facilities and health care services, planners must be able to accurately predict future health personnel needs to ensure an appropriate supply of physicians. David A. Kindig and Hormoz Movassaghi provide a comprehensive examination of the report of the Graduate Medical Education National Advisory Committee (GMENAC), which has influenced health policy during the 1980s. They examine GMENAC, as well as other studies, in terms of the strengths and limitations of their assumptions and methodologies. The authors then offer conclusions regarding specialty and geographic distribution of physicians at the beginning of the next century.

In the concluding chapter, Barbara Barzansky compares the current perceived problems and proposed changes in medical education with those of the early twentieth century and contrasts current forces acting to bring about change with those of the past. Her focus is on four recent reports originating from within the medical education community. In her analysis, she notes the relative similarity of recommendations for change, considers possible implementation strategies, and comments on the likelihood of success.

BEYOND FLEXNER

1

Abraham Flexner in Historical Perspective

Robert P. Hudson

In early 1909, with the cooperation of the American Medical Association and the sponsorship of the Carnegie Foundation for the Advancement of Teaching, an implacable little schoolmaster from Louisville, Kentucky set out on the first of 155 visits to all the medical schools in the United States and Canada. At each school he was interested in:

First, the entrance requirements. What were they? Were they enforced? Second, the size and training of the faculty. Third, the sum available from endowment and fees for the support of the institution, and what became of it. Fourth, the quality and adequacy of the laboratories provided for the instruction of the first two years and the qualifications and training of the teachers of the so-called preclinical branches. Fifth, and finally, the relations between medical schools and hospitals, including particularly freedom of access to beds and freedom in the appointment by the school of the hospital physicians and surgeons who automatically should become clinical teachers.[1]

His findings, published in 1910 and thereafter called the "Flexner Report,"[2] will be discussed in detail in what follows. In summary, his verdict was that medical education in the United States in 1910 was, quite simply, abysmal.

In the ensuing years, Abraham Flexner was both reviled and revered. Since his death in 1959, his influence has been reviewed, reappraised, reconsidered, refined, and revised. At first glance another attempt at assessing the man and his work would appear to be an exercise in pounding sand. When one gets into it, however, a genuine opportunity emerges. The corpus of analysis that has accumulated in recent years reveals how enduringly the Flexnerian presence has persisted over more than three-quarters of a century. His spirit has been accorded none of the rest ordinarily associated with shaking off the mortal coils. He has not been permitted to fulfill the definition in that wonderful little book, *The Devil's Dictionary* by Ambrose Bierce, where a corpse is defined as a "person who manifests the highest possible degree of indifference that is consistent with a civil regard for the solicitude of others."[3] It is, of course, more accurate to say that the want of indifference is ours, not Flexner's. However, his shade has become something of a poltergeist. Between intervals of decent silence we hear rappings and other unexpected noises that bring him back for new historical discussion (discussion here redefined as the historian's polite "method of confirming others in their errors").

There are two assumptions underlying this introductory essay. First, it is assumed the reader is aware that for most of the nineteenth century the proprietary form of medical education common in the United States was distinctly deficient. The second assumption is that many prospective readers are not deeply conversant with the changes that preceded the "Flexner Report," the details of the Report itself, or its immediate and long-range effects.

The one fact, perhaps the only one, upon which practically all historians now agree is that reform of American medical education was progressing on a broad front before the "Flexner Report" was published in 1910. This point requires emphasis because many educators and others retain the notion that reform in American medical education began with Flexner. This simplistic and erroneous conclusion endures despite direct statements by Flexner in the Report itself "that, especially in the last fifteen years, substantial progress has been made,"[4] and in his autobiography, where he says that "Progress had indeed begun long before my day."[5] Before examining Flexner's own contribution, some of the forces that were changing American medical education prior to 1910 are described.

FORCES FOR CHANGE IN MEDICAL EDUCATION BEFORE FLEXNER

Once long ago I analyzed the educational patterns of the 1,513 physicians listed in the *Dictionary of American Medical Biography* (*DAMB*) who completed their formal medical training in the United States during the nineteenth century.[6] This was the antediluvian period of statistical studies in which the state of the art featured cards sorted by an over-sized icepick, and calculators incapable of handling square roots. It is the sort of endeavor recommended to anyone who suffers insomnia or masochism. In short, the study provided numerical evidence, some of which is summarized below, to support the contention that significant improvements in American medical education had occurred across a broad front before the "Flexner Report."

The Educational Preparation of Physicians

The educational preparation of physicians improved as the nineteenth century progressed. More students undertook premedical education, which was itself improving as the public began to perceive the utility of high school and collegiate education, and the benefits possible from basic and applied research. Of those in the *DAMB* sample completing training in the first decade of the nineteenth century, 36 percent took undergraduate degrees before studying medicine. This is compared to 63 percent of those completing training in the last decade. Fifty-five percent of the sample earned a medical degree before entering practice in the first decade, compared to 100 percent in the last. During the century an increasing number of students constructed informal arrangements for post-doctoral clinical training, the experience we now label residency training. In the *DAMB* study, only 1.6 percent took such training in the first decade; the figure for the last decade was 44 percent.

Considering the fact that none of the educational endeavors listed above was legally imposed for most of the century, these self-generated movements are remarkable. Beyond these, another significant group studied abroad. As the century progressed more and more American students pursued additional training in Britain and France, but especially in Germany and Austria. In the *DAMB* sample the figures were 15 percent in the first decade, 36 percent in the last. To minimize the possibility that these sojourns were for enrichment other than medical education, only instances were counted in which the European experience took place within five years of the completion of American medical training.

The Impact of European Medical Education

The small numbers in the *DAMB* study do not reflect the impact of European medical education on American physicians at the time. Bonner estimated that some fifteen thousand Americans sought medical experience in Germany and Austria alone during the years 1870–1914. In his words, "What Americans found in the German university in the last half of the nineteenth century was a revelation. In organization, spirit, facilities, and productivity, the German university was reaching the zenith of its influence by 1870."[7]

The roster of professors available to these young Americans reads like a Who's Who of contemporary biomedical sciences. Not even the most inventive gerrymandering would have allowed an American student at the time to put together at home an experience paralleling that routinely available in Germany and Austria. As few of the Americans were seeking degrees, they had essentially complete freedom to wander from one center to another. This allowed them to tailor their educational experiences to their personal needs. Those seeking advanced study in the basic sciences frequently attended smaller German universities; those pursuing excellence in clinical specialties went to Berlin or Vienna, particularly the latter.

This phenomenal medical migration affected American medicine in at least three broad areas. First, many of the prominent American researchers during the fifty years after the Civil War visited Europe, and the European influence on this group and their students was profound in terms of the later elevation of research in the United States.[8]

Second, the German and Viennese clinics gave strong impetus to the rise of specialism as it began in the United States during the last half of the century. At that time, most American practitioners were hostile to the concept of specialization, and this hostility persisted in many cases up to World War II. Many rationalizations were put forth for this opposition, but the real reasons related to status and income. Rather quickly it became apparent that the individual who mastered the new ophthalmoscope or laryngoscope or who had outstanding success in orthopedic surgery earned more money and rose in public esteem. Still, for years these de facto specialists called themselves general practitioners and actually practiced a certain amount of general medicine.[9] Admitting the difficulties in accurately labeling a given individual as a specialist, the *DAMB* study still reflects the movement in broad terms. The biographies leave little doubt that many thought of themselves as specialists and limited their practices to the extent permitted by societal and collegial pressures. The chief value of the *DAMB* entries is the demonstration that specialization originated in the minds and practices of many American physicians well before the public or the profession took cognizance of the movement. The broad trend to specialism is best reflected in the *DAMB* sample by the decrease in general practitioners as the century progressed. In the first decade 87 percent were classified as generalists, but in the ninth decade only 27 percent were so classified. The sample also reveals that those classified as specialists more often took premedical degrees and postgraduate training, and engaged in study abroad. Not unexpectedly, all of these trends themselves increased decade by decade, particularly after mid-century.

The third influence of European medical institutions on American medicine was mediated through the major innovation in medical education made possible by Baltimore businessman Johns Hopkins. The Johns Hopkins School of Medicine was founded almost two decades before the "Flexner Report," and it drew directly from the best in British, French, and German institutions. In one of its first actions, the Trustees of the Johns Hopkins University invited the presidents of Harvard, Cornell, and Michigan to discuss the character of the proposed school. All three men had studied in Germany, although they did not insist that the Baltimore institution be fashioned along German lines. They were unanimous, however, in independently recommending Daniel Coit Gilman as first president of Johns Hopkins.[10] Although he never meant to recreate a German university, Gilman had visited there and had many features of the German model in mind.[11]

The Johns Hopkins School of Medicine itself became a major factor in reform, when it opened in 1893 requiring a baccalaureate degree for admission and four years of study for the medical degree. Despite gloomy predictions the experiment quickly proved that at least some American students wanted a high-quality domestic medical education.[12]

Medical School Linkages with Universities

Another major force for change in medical education was the tightening linkage between medical schools and universities. In the first half of the nineteenth century, the affiliations that existed between medical schools and universities were largely nominal. In practice the medical schools were owned by their physician-faculties and operated independently of the universities whose names lent some measure of illusory prestige to the arrangement. This changed after mid-century as the universities began to take more active control of their affiliated medical colleges. The transformation resulted from a new perception of the university itself, which pivoted on the shift to the natural sciences as sources of new knowledge and also the attempt to make the humanities more "scientific" in their endeavor and purpose. As the proliferation of knowledge accelerated and began to exhibit its potential, the university became its functional locus. By the last quarter of the nineteenth century, some universities in keeping with their new and broader mission set out to upgrade their medical branches, and those universities lacking medical schools began actively creating them. As Ludmerer has emphasized, the post-Civil War universities saw their duty as creating new knowledge as well as preserving the old, and challenging dogma rather than merely defending it. This new outlook spread to the medical faculties as well, and gradually yet inevitably the earlier nominal ties between university and medical school became real and important to the mutual benefit of both parties.[13]

Re-Appearance of Legislative Control of Medical Practice

Another important element in the pre-Flexnerian period was the absence of legislative control of medical practice. At the end of the third decade of the nineteenth century, most states had laws governing licensure. After about 1830 the states began repealing these laws, thus ending the putative monopoly enjoyed by "regular" physicians at the time. Reginald Fitz attributed the beginnings of this movement to the rise of one of the more successful early medical sects, the Thomsonians. In reality the sectarian movement, rather than causal in this regard, emerged into the vacuum of legal control that came about as the states abdicated regulation of medical licensure.[14]

Curiously, from the 1830s until around 1875, legislative regulation of medicine was eschewed by all involved.[15] State lawmakers shunned it as class legislation and saw the "regular" physician as seeking a monopoly. Regular physicians objected on grounds that the proposed laws, in the very regulation of sectarians, implied recognition and conferred protection. The public, for its part, would tolerate no interference in the right of every citizen to choose a medical attendant. From 1840 on there was growing public dissatisfaction with the dogmatic adherence by the "regulars" to their regimen of bloodletting, purging, emetics, and other "evacuants," which, for good reason, came to be known as "heroic therapy."[16] Later, with westward expansion and the rapid increase in population, low standards were justified on the basis of the unique "genius and habits" of the American people. The spirit of Jacksonian democracy affected medical practice, as well as many other institutions of the time.[17]

Pressure from National Medical Organizations

Revitalized national medical organizations also contributed to nineteenth-century reform. Perhaps "vitalized" would be a better term, since neither the American Medical Association (AMA) nor what came to be called the Association of American Medical Colleges (AAMC) enjoyed effective life until late in the nineteenth century.

The AMA, which had educational reform as a principal raison d'etre from its beginnings in 1846, could do little in the following years beyond mounting a steady drumbeat of editorial lamentations in its journal. In part this was due to a factional split that existed from the AMA's origin. Luring the physician-owners of the proprietary schools into an organization committed to reforming those same schools would require that they be given disproportionately large voting power. But to give the medical colleges an inordinate voice would subvert all efforts at change. The compromise was flawed from the outset. Only a third or so of eligible medical schools were represented at the AMA's organizational meeting in 1846. By 1853 the split was so hopeless that there was a move to exclude the medical college delegates altogether. The best that can be said for the AMA before 1900 is that its efforts did keep reform vaguely alive in the distant hollows of the profession's conscience.[18]

In 1904 the AMA established a standing Council on Medical Education, which periodically inspected and rated the medical schools. From that point on the AMA's long-muted voice finally began to be heard. In 1908 the Council enlisted the Carnegie Foundation in support of Flexner's survey. The data accumulated from previous AMA inspections were made available to Flexner and undoubtedly contributed to the effectiveness of the whirlwind inspections for which Flexner was later criticized.

In 1876 representatives of twenty-two medical colleges answered a call to explore possibilities for reform from within academe itself. Organized the following year as the American Medical College Association, the reformers fell on hard times and ultimate self-destruction after voting to require three years of medical training, lasting at least six months each year, in an approved medical college. In 1890 a successful reorganization took place, and from 1896 on, the AAMC played an increasingly influential role through its unrelenting pressures for higher admission standards and more rigorous requirements for the medical degree.[19]

OUTCOMES OF THE FLEXNER REPORT

To this point we have seen that before Abraham Flexner began his survey in 1909, reform of medical education was already underway in a number of areas. Given this, it is fair to ask why the "Flexner Report" maintains its lofty position; why, for example, was it considered sufficiently prestigious to be included in a 1974 issue of *Daedalus* entitled "Twentieth-Century Classics Revisited."[20]

Curiously, the "Flexner Report" became a classic in part because it was consistently misunderstood. This related to the fact that it was more often cited than read. For many, including academics, the "Flexner Report" is still seen as the document that singlehandedly called public and professional attention to the sorry state of American medical education, and produced the dramatic contrast between the scene in 1850 and that of a century later. The misreadings of Flexner's essay are apparent in the myths that came to enshroud his report.

But misconceptions alone do not account for the Report's inclusion in *Daedalus*. The scholars making the selection for this issue were given complete freedom to choose their entries, and it was not a misunderstanding of the Report that led Carleton Chapman to select it for *Daedalus*. Brieger is correct in saying the Report is a classic, not in the sense that it invites rereading for sheer enjoyment and profit, but because it ranks high among books that stimulated "profound social changes." Flexner's "genteel bombshell," as it has been termed, was a classic of muckraking literature in the best sense of that genre. It may not have been revolutionary, but it "proved highly influential, along with Michael Harrington's *The Other America*, which stimulated the great society programs of the 1960s, Betty Friedan's *The Feminine Mystique*, Rachel Carson's *The Silent Spring*, and Ralph Nader's *Unsafe At Any Speed.*"[21]

One way to assess the effects of the "Flexner Report" is to compare the seven major recommendations made by Flexner with the actual events that occurred in medical education. Two of the seven recommendations can be dealt with as one. The first was that the number of poorly trained physicians be cut, and the second was that the number of medical schools be reduced from 155 to 31.[22] This linkage was a natural one. Long before Flexner there were too many schools for the pool of qualified applicants. Competition had reduced standards for admission and graduation to far less than an ideal minimum. As a consequence, too many poorly trained physicians were being produced. Whether too many physicians per se were being turned out is a different question. What is certain is that the number of medical colleges declined during the period under discussion, and as noted, this movement was underway before the "Flexner Report" appeared. In part due to the inspections and ratings of the Council on Medical Education of the AMA that began in 1906, twenty-nine schools merged or closed between 1906 and 1910. By 1910, 131 schools survived, but this number decreased steadily to ninety-six in 1915, eighty-five in 1920, eighty in 1925, and seventy-six in 1930.[23]

Flexner's ideal of thirty-one schools was never approached but the figures above suggest that significant progress occurred. In fact, while the number of schools declined, the numbers of graduates did not decrease proportionately. For each fifth year beginning with 1910, graduates numbered 4,440, 3,536, 3,047, 3,974, and 4,565.[24] Had nothing really changed? The numbers of schools and graduates alone do not give the whole picture. True, the number of graduates in 1930 actually exceeded those of 1910, but a more important figure, the physician-population ratio, did decline. The number of physicians per 100,000 population over the decades in question were: 1900–157, 1910–164, 1920–137, 1930–125, 1940–126, and 1950–134.[25] The problems of interpreting such figures for periods separated by a century are obvious, but the ratios at least raise a question concerning Flexner's contention that too many physicians were being produced for the current and future needs of the country. N. S. Davis calculated that physicians and population increased at an equal rate in the thirty-five years before 1876.[26] Stern estimated the physician-population ratio at 1:572 in 1860 and 1:578 in 1900.[27] Flexner agreed with Stern, but simply argued that the ratio was too large.[28] Later trends raise questions about Flexner's conclusion, at least in terms of public perception and policy. By 1982 the ratio was 1:460.[29] These figures do not demonstrate that Flexner's recommendation was wrong for his time, only that society apparently disagreed with it as long-term projection. Better physicians were needed, not necessarily fewer. For Flexner, the way to increase quality was to decrease numbers.

Flexner's next contention was that premedical education required a level of scientific understanding not obtainable from a high school education alone. He perceived that the basic sciences of medical school, anatomy, physiology, and what we now term biochemistry, were second-level sciences; that is, they required a solid background in biology, chemistry, and physics. The facts did not support the assumption that students entered medical school with this background. Not only were high schools deficient in this regard, but in general colleges themselves were not sufficiently demanding. Not only was the quality of high school and collegiate preparation lacking but the medical schools required too little premedical study, however deficient. In a chapter entitled "The Actual Basis of Medical Education," Flexner detailed the prevailing situation. Only sixteen institutions required two or more years of college preparation; about fifty required nothing beyond a four-year high school education or its "equivalent," a term Flexner derided by denoting it as a "device that concedes the necessity of a standard which it forthwith proceeds to evade." The remainder of medical schools demanded nothing more than a common school education.[30] At a minimum, he believed, premedical preparation should consist of two years of college with heavy emphasis on the sciences.

In Flexner's view, even this improvement would not suffice for long. The physician's role was changing from curing individual patients to a broader, socially-oriented emphasis on prevention. For this physicians would require more than a solid scientific knowledge base; they must be educated persons in the broader sense of the word.[31]

Improvement in premedical education was slow in coming. By 1925 Flexner observed that only a few medical schools required three or more years of college preparation.[32] Even then collegiate standards were so lax and variable that "the physician is only occasionally an educated man."[33]

Lamentations regarding the inadequacies of premedical education have reappeared since the "Flexner Report" with a dismal regularity that is reminiscent of the AMA's mournful editorials between 1847 and 1904. One of the latest of this ilk is *Physicians for the Twenty-First Century* published in 1984.[34] Once again the same plea is made. All we need, these reports seem to tell us, is an educational system that will provide medical school admissions committees with a generous pool of applicants who are inherently humane, broadly-educated, socially-aware, essentially philanthropic, and soundly based in the biologic and physical sciences.

Flexner also argued that medical practitioners should be scientists in terms of treating each new clinical encounter as an exercise in scientific inquiry. This led to one of the most serious misreadings of the "Flexner

Report," the notion that research and science were more important than medical practice. As Flexner saw it, science must underpin the patient workup, and new knowledge might follow such an approach. But this did not mean that every physician was to be a researcher in the usual meaning of the word. The quest for new knowledge should not dwarf endeavors to heal the ill; that is, research should not occur at the expense of the practice of medicine. For Flexner investigation and practice were "one in spirit, method, and object."[35] That one physician should pass a life emphasizing investigation while another engaged chiefly in practice was merely a division of emphasis and labor, not a division in the basic nature of their activities.

On this point, Flexner's ideal was nearly achieved. Gradually the medical workup, particularly as supported by the objectivity of laboratory medicine, assumed something of the nature of a scientific inquiry. A number of physicians, particularly but not exclusively in academic settings, collectivized the process into what came to be called clinical research. Gradually, new discoveries put the process on an increasingly scientific basis and physicians became inordinately disease-oriented. As they realized Flexner's ideal of making each new patient encounter an exercise in scientific inquiry, physicians neglected the ancient emphasis on the patient as person. This transgression ranks high among the reasons for the profession's decline in stature in recent years.[36]

Flexner's fifth suggestion was that most, but not necessarily all, faculty members should engage in research. There is no doubt that he saw strong redemptive features in first-hand research. At one point he says without exception that "research is required of the medical faculty because only research will keep the teachers in condition."[37] But Flexner was always aware of what was possible at the moment. In the late nineteenth and early twentieth centuries Americans were only beginning to rebel at their longstanding dependence on European science and to perceive the practical as well as theoretical advantages of a "home-grown" science. What little support existed for research derived from private philanthropy, not state or federal funding. So that Flexner, soon after the unequivocal statement just quoted, goes on to say, "On the other hand, it will never happen that every professor in either the medical school or the university faculty is a genuinely productive scientist. There is room for men of another type, the non-productive, assimilative teacher of wide learning, continuous receptivity, critical sense, and responsive interest."[38]

Despite Flexner's qualification, the idea that all medical academicians must be researchers, either basic or clinical, became dominant. A slide that brought appreciative snickers at medical meetings in the 1960s showed Christ on the cross above a caption that read, "He was a great healer and teacher but He just didn't publish."

A trend toward division of labor developed, that is, non-physicians taught in the basic sciences and physicians in the clinical years. This separation already existed when Flexner surveyed his surroundings. In the decades immediately after the Civil War, basic science teaching and most basic medical research was done by physicians. After 1890 or so the numbers of nonmedical graduate students increased at an astonishing rate.[39] This was the movement that eventually transferred most basic science teaching and much basic research to Ph.D.s. By Flexner's time it was still an innovation to be "watched with interest,"[40] but the trend was inexorable. By the 1960s the physician-basic scientist was an esoteric hybrid.

Flexner's sixth recommendation was that medical schools must control hospital beds for purposes of clinical instruction. The vast majority of nineteenth-century medical schools had no genuine working relationship with a hospital, thus no opportunities for bedside teaching in the modern sense. With a few notable exceptions, ante-bellum clinical instruction took place in classrooms and amphitheaters. Even the fact of an affiliation between medical school and hospital did not guarantee the student access to patients. The preceptorship was devised to remedy this deficiency, and in theory could have done so. In fact, the arrangement was rather loose even in its inception, and deteriorated along with other standards of education as the century progressed. In many instances it became perfunctory. The student paid the required fee, had essentially no exposure to the preceptor, and picked up his certificate at the end of two or three years. Flexner realized that in an open and unregulated educational marketplace, the preceptorship alone could never provide the requisite clinical experience. Thus, for him the only solution was genuine control of teaching beds by university-affiliated medical schools.

In Flexner's mind, the emerging dispute over which facts—those from the laboratory or those from the bedside—were more important for patient care was senseless. In one situation laboratory data might be more useful, in another the findings at the bedside. Often the best approach integrated the two types of data.[41] But again ideal amalgamation could be effected only if the medical school controlled its hospital beds. "The student can never be part of the organization in a hospital in which he is present on sufferance." And, Flexner went on to argue, the same could be said of the faculty.[42]

By about 1900 numerous influential observers saw the chief obstacle to improving medical education as obtaining access to good teaching hospitals. During the first decades of the twentieth century few could build their own teaching hospitals, which was felt to be the ideal solution.

Many found the road to affiliation with existing hospitals pocked with potholes. Trustees of private hospitals had difficulty seeing that the quid pro quo of affiliation justified the bother.[43] Despite all obstacles, the twenty or so years after the "Flexner Report" witnessed the rise of the teaching hospital. Some were built with public monies, but most derived from a new symbiosis between the medical schools and existing public and private hospitals.[44]

In summary, the evolution of clinical teaching in the United States was an uneven process. The beginning was promising; the first medical school in the nation began operating in 1765 as the Medical Department of the University of Pennsylvania. From its inception it recognized the importance of a clinical affiliation, which began in the fall of 1766 when Thomas Bond began a series of clinical lectures at the Pennsylvania Hospital.[45] But this salutary movement, with other sound educational endeavors, foundered during the proprietary period. A revival gained momentum during the last quarter of the nineteenth century, but sound, systematic clinical teaching was not generally in place until some 165 years after Bond's tentative efforts.

Flexner's last major recommendation was that state regulation of medical licensure should be strengthened. As noted, from about 1830 until after the Civil War, state regulation of medical education and practice was all but abandoned. By 1875 the resultant chaos no longer could be ignored. The states reversed their earlier policies and began writing new laws governing licensure and practice.[46] By 1894 Fitz could report that all states except New Hampshire and Massachusetts had some form of legislative control of medical practice. Not unexpectedly the laws varied widely in intent and prosecution, but Fitz concluded that "to them, more than any one cause, is due the difference which exists between the condition now and in 1870."[47] Thus, the movement toward state regulation was already well underway when Flexner predicted in 1910 that "The state boards are the instruments through which the reconstruction of medical education will be largely effected."[48]

The impact of the "Flexner Report" has been widely disputed with opinions ranging from "almost no effect" to the conclusion that it produced a revolution in American medical education.[49] In a strict sense Ludmerer is correct in saying that, "Conceptually, Flexner's discussion of proper medical teaching contained no new ideas."[50] But what it did contain was names and places, with disgraceful conditions starkly revealed. There is no doubt that the Report led many faculties, legislators, and others to examine their institutions as they never had before. Simply to show that all or most of Flexner's recommendations were spottily in place before the Report does not mean that the Report had little effect. On the contrary, the widespread public interest following the journalistic response to the Report had significant immediate and long-range effects.

Having digested most of the assessment of the past fifteen years, I am still prepared to stand on my original general impression that "Flexner's contribution was not so much revolutionary as catalytic to an already evolving process."[51] That it produced headlines across the nation, lawsuits, and even a threat on Flexner's life does not alter the fact that changes had already taken place which simply were not widely recognized at the time.

REASONS FOR THE IMPORTANCE OF THE FLEXNER REPORT

If the Report was largely catalytic rather than innovative, the question remains: how did it achieve its mythic proportions? In Chapman's view there were three reasons. First, it came at precisely the right time. Second, due in significant parts to Flexner's own efforts, money was forthcoming to bring a number of other schools up to the standards of Johns Hopkins, the school that Flexner held as a model. Finally, the Report stood alone in saying what other would-be reformers wanted to say but could not.[52] Regarding the latter, mention has been made of the increasing importance after 1904 of the AMA's Council on Medical Education through its inspection and ratings of medical schools, its request to the Carnegie Foundation that contributed to the decision to undertake an objective outside look at the nation's medical schools, and its provision of its inspection data to Flexner, who was also accompanied on many of his visits by N. P. Colwell, the Council's secretary. Still, it must be remembered that the Council had a fine line to walk. The AMA at the time probably represented fewer than ten percent of the nation's physicians. In addition the Council was an elite group with strong leanings to research and academic excellence. The AMA was a numerical minority among the nation's physicians, and the Council, in many ways, was a philosophical minority within the AMA itself. Thus, in the view of Arthur Dean Bevan, chairman of the Council, the AMA might achieve its long-standing goal of educational reform by using Flexner and the Carnegie Foundation as stalking horses.[53]

In raising money for medical education, Abraham Flexner had no peers. As but one example of his direct effect, in 1920 Flexner helped persuade George Eastman to give five million dollars to create the University of Rochester School of Medicine. Through his position on the General Education Board of the Rockefeller Foundation, Flexner presided over the distribution of some fifty million dollars. As Flexner had anticipated, this philanthropy stimulated a new and healthier competition among the nation's medical schools. When one school received funds from the Rockefeller Foundation, others sought their own philanthropy

or began to convince taxpayers of the benefits to be derived from supporting their state medical schools.[54]

The issue of money raises another interpretation of the Flexner era
that has appeared in recent years. This is the Marxist interpretation put
forth by Howard Berliner, E. Richard Brown and others, which centers
on the motives of Flexner, the Rockefeller and Carnegie Foundations,
and others whose philanthropy supported reform in medical education
at the time.[55] The story is too complex for full explication here, but
neither can it justly be ignored. Berliner concludes that the AMA supported the "Flexner Report" to eliminate the competing medical sects
of the period. He contends that the licensing boards of the period were
effectively controlled by AMA members and that the examination questions were designed to discriminate against students training in the "non-
scientific" schools. It may appear strange that he would fault the reformers because they favored students trained in the more scientific
schools, but the reader must understand that Berliner sees little merit
in the changes effected by the new science in medicine. He apparently
arrives at this conclusion by pointing to recent commentators such as
McKeown, who argues that the principal victories over infectious diseases
resulted not from direct physician intervention but from improvements
in general hygiene and nutrition.[56] Berliner seems not to understand
that even though improvements in hygiene and nutrition were underway
by the last quarter of the nineteenth century, the new bacteriology and
biochemistry placed the improvements on a scientific basis on which all
could agree and thus gave them tremendous impetus. Berliner chooses
to downplay the remarkable gains in understanding and treating diseases
that resulted from the new science. It is true that great benefit derived
from a general cleansing of the environment, but it took the new bacteriology to tell the rural family how to avoid typhoid fever by a judicious
juxtaposition of their water well and outhouse, and why their milk should
be pasteurized. Granted, health was bound to be improved by more
food; still it required biochemistry to establish the notion of "better"
food, and to elucidate the entire category of deficiency diseases.

Having established, in his mind, a licensure system dominated by sci-
entifically-oriented members of the AMA, Berliner naturally concludes
that the AMA supported the "Flexner Report" in order to eliminate
competing sectarians. Members of the licensing boards would simply
construct requirements that favored the scientific candidates over the
non-scientific allopathic candidates and the sectarians. How he can find
only capitalistic conspiracy and no redemption in this movement can be
clear only to the historian who shares Berliner's inherent bias. Further
evidence of this historical "tunnel vision" is found in his conclusion that
the Carnegie Foundation supported the "Flexner Report," and the Rockefeller Foundation implemented it, to create good will for capitalism;

and that medicine was perceived by Gates, for example, as "not just a means of improving health, but a means of ameliorating class struggle."[57]

For several years, without making any serious analysis of my reaction to Marxist-oriented medical history, I was vaguely bothered by the approach. I am indebted to Daniel Fox for clarifying my thoughts on the matter. While he grants the Marxists a definite heuristic value, Fox ultimately rejects all monolithic approaches to history, asserting that, "Neat hypotheses—whether they derive from Marxism, liberal pluralism, Christian faith or some other commitment—give me aesthetic pleasure. But I suspect my delight. History is too complicated to remain for very long 'explained' by any hypothesis."[58]

I agree with Fox, and concerning reform in medical education a good comparison with Berliner is Ludmerer's *Learning to Heal*. One cannot read Ludmerer without concluding that even before Flexner, at several medical schools in the United States, there were faculty members who advocated reform because they believed in it as a matter of principle and who engaged in altruistic behavior that was not in their economic self-interest. They saw reducing the number of schools and the size of classes as the only way to raise standards, and not as some larger scheme by the AMA to eliminate sectarianism and reduce the number of physicians, thereby eliminating competition.[59]

It can be argued that even though it was against their immediate economic interests, these reformers benefited professionally in terms of academic advancement, the gratification of leadership roles, and the general trappings of public recognition, all of which would benefit their economic interests indirectly. This contention is ultimately irrefutable because motivation is often hidden even from the individual involved. It is possible that human beings are incapable of pure altruism, and that we may have to settle for the good that comes from those who manage to be more selfless than selfish. The alternative is to fall back on Bierce's cousin, H. L. Mencken, whose appeal derives from the fact that his cynicism is so hyperbolically pure, and who wrote on one occasion, "A show of altruism is respected chiefly for selfish motives. Everyone figures himself profiting by it tomorrow."[60]

Another area where Berliner disagrees with Flexner relates to the "poor boy" argument. Proprietary schools argued that some medical schools which were inadequate according to Flexner's standards because they could not modernize their curriculums or facilities should be preserved so that students without much money could attend. The charge was made by some that Flexner's ideal medical school would effectively prevent poor students from obtaining a medical education. Flexner disagreed, believing that second-rate medical schools would result in second-rate physicians. Berliner says, "Of all the changes that have ensued in medicine since the publication of the "Flexner Report" in 1910, the change in class composition of the medical labor force has been the most significant."[61] The statement is at least arguable as it stands, but even if it is accepted, surely few would argue that abominable medical education should have been preserved so the poor boy could become a poor physician. Berliner seems to acknowledge the existence of a problem by gently taking Flexner to task because he did not recommend a scholarship program for poor students. In this context, it should be mentioned that Flexner realized his suggestions were meant for the present. His was no plan for the ages, as he made clear in his caveat, "In the course of the next thirty years needs will develop of which we here take no account. As we cannot foretell them, we shall not endeavor to meet them."[62]

MYTHS RELATED TO THE FLEXNER REPORT

A number of historians have described the myths that have accrued to the "Flexner Report" over the years. Gert Brieger produced the best such summary in the inaugural issue of *Medical Heritage*.[63] Many writers claim that the Report has been misconstrued because so few have actually read it. In fact, so many commentators have made this point that if they themselves have read it, the Report has reached some sort of audience. Brieger extends this point by emphasizing that a number of myths came about because commentators limited their reading of Flexner to the Report alone, ignoring his voluminous other writings as well as those of persons associated closely with him.

One Flexnerian myth is that his visits to the schools were too short to permit an accurate assessment. A careful reading of Flexner's descriptions of his methods, as well as analyses by others, convinces me that he could arrive at reasonably accurate conclusions. This does not deny that other considerations such as politics influenced his conclusions and actions at times, as Pat Ward has shown in the case of Chicago.[64]

Perhaps, the most telling example of Flexner's efficiency is the story, which has been detailed by Munger and others, of Robert Brookings at Washington University of St. Louis. Before Flexner's visit Brookings had given faithful guidance and financial support to the medical school. In a letter to Henry Pritchett, president of the Carnegie Foundation, Brookings took strong exception to Flexner's short visit and unfavorable assessment. Flexner revisited St. Louis, took Brookings along on a reinspection, and convinced him of the miserable reality of the original evaluation.[65]

Also, for the most part, the schools of Flexner's time were extremely simple by today's standards; and current accreditation site visits are relatively short. For example, in 1986 the Kansas University Medical School had an annual operating budget of 170 million dollars, a full-time faculty of 560, clinical facilities in both Kansas City and Wichita, and affiliations with another half-dozen hospitals. The 1986 Liaison Committee on Medical Education accreditation visit for this school took only a bit more than three days.

A second widespread misconception is that Flexner advocated the lockstep curriculum that became characteristic of schools as they reformed according to the Johns Hopkins model.[66] Why this perception arose is fascinating, since it is totally contrary to Flexner's stated views. The obvious though not necessarily complete explanation is that Flexner's Report and his other writings simply were not read. Because he extolled the Johns Hopkins Medical School as the best *at the time*, and because the medical colleges gradually locked themselves into this model due to its perceived merit, the unexamined and erroneous assumption was that Flexner believed the Hopkins model should become universal. Flexner's writings and actions both before and after publication of the Report support the contention that this conclusion is false. His preparatory school in Louisville was flexible in the extreme. In his words, "The school was operated without rules, without examinations, without records, and without reports."[67] Students progressed according to their demonstrated abilities. Certainly the Institute for Advanced Study, which Flexner later helped found and then headed, was based on the importance of individual creativity and academic flexibility.[68] Finally, in his 1925 book on comparative medical education, he excoriated the lockstep curriculum, by then ubiquitous, saying, "Anything more alien to the spirit of scientific or modern medicine or to university life could hardly be contrived."[69]

Brieger considers a third myth the most significant, namely that the Report "stressed research and science at the expense of the practice of medicine." Flexner did not believe that practitioners were unimportant. On the contrary he felt they were a vital part of the medical scene. However, their practice had to be based on science, and each patient should be approached with the same rigorous thinking and methods that characterized a scientific exercise. This misunderstanding as Brieger emphasizes, "led to much fruitless discussion of science *versus* the art of medicine, when all along we should have been speaking of science *and* art."[70]

FLEXNER'S CONTRIBUTIONS TO MEDICAL EDUCATION

Earlier commentators have differed widely about Flexner's contribution to the reform of medical education. This diversity of opinion will continue. In *Learning To Heal*, Ludmerer states that, "Contrary to popular perception, neither Abraham Flexner nor the American Medical Association participated in the creation of modern American medical education." His point is that the concepts that came to characterize the new medical education were already being tested at various schools before 1904 when the AMA Council on Medical Education was formed or 1910 when the "Flexner Report" appeared. Ludmerer does agree that Flexner and the AMA "profoundly influenced the final form that the system took."[71] A great deal here hangs on what Ludmerer means by the phrase "participated in the creation of modern American medical education." If he means only that the ideas that characterized the form of modern medical education were not original or even wholly subscribed to by Flexner and spokesmen for the AMA, his position is defensible. But to some that use of the phrase may be too restrictive. Ludmerer demonstrates that a few medical schools were experimenting with the reforms under discussion and that one, John Hopkins, had brought many of the concepts together in practice. But conception and implementation on a small scale would not necessarily lead to the creation of modern medical education on a national scale. An automotive society in our country was not created solely by solving the conceptual problems of the internal combustion engine or even by implementation in a few prototypes. Among many other factors, Henry Ford's assembly line played a role.

One can argue, as Ludmerer does, that reform would have occurred without Flexner. As mentioned at the outset, however, Flexner's accomplishment, which relied heavily on the AMA at its inception, had much to do with shaping public opinion and certainly accelerated the rate of change. In addition, Flexner, working through Gates, gave selected faculties an opportunity to put the pre-existing ideas to work on a broad scale long before this would otherwise have been possible. Whether or not this is participating in creation becomes, at bottom, a matter of semantic emphasis. Certainly it is the sort of historiographic analysis that prevents the continuing examination of Flexner and his times from becoming a mere exercise in pounding sand.

2

The Growth and Divergence of the Basic Sciences

Barbara Barzansky

In 1953, George Packer Berry, then dean of the Harvard Medical School, wrote:

Today's generation of doctors as they enter medical practice find a very different environment from that prevailing 50 years ago. The whole atmosphere has changed, yet the medical curriculum has not evolved to meet these changes. On the contrary, the curriculum continues to adhere to a pattern that was designed in different times and under different circumstances.[1]

Applying this criticism to the basic science portion of the curriculum, one may agree or disagree. Certainly, the specific content that is taught in the sciences has changed dramatically since the beginning of the century. However, the pattern, that is, the subjects taught, their curricular placement, and the methods used to teach them, has remained relatively constant from the early 1900s to the present.

This curricular stability is in contrast to the striking reorganization that occurred during the last quarter of the nineteenth century. In 1876, most schools offered all subjects simultaneously, and students repeated the same courses (and the same lectures) during the second year of the two-year program. Over the next twenty-five years, the curriculum moved from repetitional to graded, that is, basic science subjects came to be presented before clinical subjects. In addition, the length of medical school increased from two to three and then to four years. By 1900 nearly all medical schools had a four-year graded curriculum, with the time divided approximately equally between basic science and clinical disciplines.[2]

Abraham Flexner defined the sciences basic to medicine as anatomy (including histology and embryology), physiology (including physiological/biological chemistry), pharmacology, pathology, and bacteriology.

These, he felt, built upon the more fundamental disciplines of biology, chemistry, and physics. According to Flexner, knowledge of these fundamental sciences should be acquired before entrance to medical school, because there was no room to accommodate them in the medical curriculum.[3]

The purpose of this chapter is to trace the evolution of the basic science portion of the curriculum from the time of the "Flexner Report" to the present. This includes the amount of curricular time devoted to the basic sciences, the content taught, and the instructional formats utilized. While the medical curriculum often is described as being divided into two basic science (preclinical) and two clinical years, a number of subjects other than the traditional basic sciences have entered the first two years of the medical education program. It now is common to include topics from the behavioral and social sciences; an introduction to preventive medicine, epidemiology, and biostatistics; the fundamentals of medical ethics; and courses to teach basic clinical skills (such as interviewing and physical diagnosis).[4] The presence of these subjects in the "basic science" years affects the amount of time available for teaching the sciences, and also may affect the way content is organized in this part of the curriculum.

The teaching of the basic sciences will be examined here at fifteen-year intervals from 1910 to 1985. For each period, the general structure of the basic science curriculum will be described. In addition, excerpts from major studies or reports will be used to identify problems perceived by medical educators, and the solutions that they proposed.

Several themes are used as organizing principles. The first concerns the proper degree of integration of the basic sciences and clinical subjects. Should the basic sciences be taught as independent disciplines or should their relevance in the practice of medicine be stressed? A related theme is the appropriate educational background of basic science faculty members. Should teachers have medical training in addition to knowledge of their specific disciplines? A third theme is how to manage the steadily increasing knowledge in the basic sciences and mitigate curricular overcrowding. What guidelines should determine how much and what to teach? An examination of these themes should answer the question of how much the basic sciences have diverged from Flexner's initial conception and what forces led to this divergence.

THE FLEXNER MODEL

To Flexner, the medicine of his time was "part and parcel of modern science." The way a researcher approached a scientific problem and the way a physician approached a patient were identical—observation leading to hypothesis leading to action. The same mental qualities were needed. Therefore, the sciences and the associated scientific methods fit into the education of all physicians, whether they would eventually be general practitioners or specialists and researchers.[5]

The pedagogical framework for "modern" medical education should be active student learning. For the sciences, a purely didactic presentation was "hopelessly antiquated," belonging to "an age of accepted dogma or supposedly complete information, when the professor knew and the students learned."[6] The medical teachers in this new age might be researchers, who carried into the work of "routine instruction . . . the rigor and vigor of their research moments." In addition, there was a place for individuals of another type, "the non-productive, assimilative teacher of wide learning, continuous receptivity, critical sense, and responsive interest." However, there was no room in medical education for "the scientifically dead practitioner, whose knowledge has long since come to a standstill and whose lectures, composed when he first took his chair, like pebbles rolling in a brook, get smoother and smoother as the stream of time washes over them."[7]

Flexner approached the controversy whether or not to include clinical applications while teaching the basic sciences with a disclaimer: "a layman hesitates to offer an opinion where doctors disagree." He did argue that "medical education is a technical or professional discipline," which "calls for the possession of certain portions of many sciences arranged and organized with a distinct practical purpose in view." That purpose allows the selection of content from among the sciences, so that the parts are "organically combined." Medical education ought to be "explicitly conscious of its professional end and aim," because that is the only way that sciences can be "thoroughly kneaded." Flexner felt that teaching the basic sciences in the context of their eventual clinical application had become discredited in the United States because unqualified teachers had turned such application into a mechanical drill. Teachers with "abundant scientific knowledge and spirit" could present clinical applications without losing sight of the main educational objective.[8]

Another theme in Flexner concerned curricular diversity and flexibility.

A uniform or fixed apportion between various subjects is in schools of the highest grade neither feasible nor desirable. The endeavor to improve medical education through iron-clad prescription of curriculum or hours is a wholly mistaken effort.[9]

This approach to maintaining standards would not improve poor schools and could hinder good ones.

In summary, the Flexner model included training in the scientific method supported by active student learning. This meant abundant use of the laboratory in all basic science disciplines. More passive modes, including lectures and textbook assignments, were aids to supplement what could be learned through laboratory experiences.[10]

THE BASIC SCIENCE CURRICULUM IN 1910

A model medical curriculum developed by a committee of leading educators (Committee of One Hundred) under the auspices of the American Medical Association (AMA) Council on Medical Education was released in 1909. Of the 4,100 hours in this model curriculum, 1,970 (48 percent) were occupied by the basic sciences. In actuality, about one-fifth of the hours in the four-year curriculum were devoted to anatomy (an average of about 600–800 hours), 450 hours to physiology and biochemistry (in the best schools), 150 hours to pharmacology, and 500 hours to pathology and bacteriology. However, despite the general introduction of the graded curriculum and the lengthening of the educational program, there were significant differences in curricular hours among medical schools in 1910. For example, anatomy, which had been allotted 700 total hours in the 1909 model curriculum, ranged from 420 to 1,448 hours in U.S. medical schools.[11]

One major reason for the differences in curricular hours among schools was the amount of content from the fundamental sciences (basic biology, chemistry, and physics) that was included. For example, data in the "Flexner Report" showed that about 20 percent of the curricular hours in the first year were devoted to fundamental subjects in a medical school that required college-level science courses for entrance. At a medical school where there were only nominal admission requirements, about half of the first year was occupied by the fundamental sciences.[12]

The modern plan of course organization had appeared by the early part of the twentieth century. Concentration teaching, where students studied a small number of subjects at one time, was becoming the standard. For example, in 1899 the Harvard curriculum was reorganized with anatomy and histology/embryology in the first half of the first year, physiology and physiological (biological) chemistry in the second half of the first year, and bacteriology and pathology in the first half of the second year. Students were examined in each set of subjects before the next set began. The main advantage of the system was felt to be the student's ability to focus. Criticisms included lack of correlation among subjects, lack of opportunity for review leading to lower retention, and monotony leading to lower interest and enthusiasm.[13]

Introduction of teaching in the laboratory was arguably the major basic science innovation during the era of curriculum reform. The laboratory met Flexner's requirements for active learning. He believed that "after a strenuous laboratory discipline, the student will be ignorant of many things, but at any rate he will respect facts: he will have learned how to obtain them and what to do with them when he has them."[14] While on paper the curriculums of medical schools appeared similar, it was in the amount and quality of laboratory teaching that they differed most markedly.

Flexner recognized three categories of medical schools in his 1910 report: (1) those that required two or more years of college for entry, (2) those that required graduation from a four-year high school or the equivalent, and (3) those that had only nominal admission requirements. In the first category, the fundamental subjects had mostly disappeared from the curriculum. In the ideal circumstances, the laboratories were open all day, were well-equipped, and the professors, engaged in their own research, were always available. Some of the schools in the second category and those in the third category had laboratory facilities that were described by Flexner in scathing terms.[15]

Anatomy serves as a good example. At some schools there was no dissection. At others

dissecting rooms are indeed found, but the conditions in them defy description. The smell is intolerable; the cadavers now putrid (or) dry as tanned leather. At the Barnes Medical College (St. Louis) the (first-year students) are not permitted to dissect because first year men 'only hack and butcher.' The dissecting room of the Kansas Medical College, Topeka did duty incidentally as a chicken yard: corn was scattered over the floor—along with other things—and the poultry fed placidly in the long intervals before instruction in anatomy began.[16]

There were equally damning comments about the poor quality of facilities and laboratory instruction in the other basic science disciplines.

Leading medical educators accepted the importance of laboratory teaching. A 1910 model medical curriculum proposed by the Committee on Curriculum of the Association of American Medical Colleges (AAMC) allotted 2,010 hours (about half of the total 4,000 hours) to the basic sciences. Of the basic science hours, 61 percent were allotted to the laboratory. Incidentally, this model curriculum closely resembles the curriculum proposed by the AMA Council on Medical Education's Committee of One Hundred, indicating that there was consensus among the academic leadership about how the medical education program should be organized.[17]

Opposing viewpoints on whether to stress the clinical relevance of the basic sciences and whether teachers should have medical training were being advanced at this time. One side of the argument can be summarized by stating the opinions of Dr. William Welch (founding dean of the Johns Hopkins Medical School) and Dr. Arthur Dean Bevan (first chair of the AMA Council on Medical Education). In an article titled "The Medical Curriculum," Welch asked the question, "What is the object of medical education?" His answer was unequivocal, the purpose was

to make good doctors. There is no question that this should be the underlying conception in our schemes for medical education, and unless you can define a given course as bearing on that training, it has no place in the medical curriculum. If the training in physiology cannot be shown to make good doctors, it is not defensible.[18]

Bevan was equally certain that teachers of the basic sciences would be better for having medical training. In the absence of properly trained physicians, many positions in the basic sciences were filled by individuals with Ph.D. degrees. While Bevan felt that these individuals were able,

all of them would be much better fitted for teaching in a medical school if, in addition to their special training, they had completed a medical course including one year of hospital work. This training would give them the medical point of view and place them in a position where they could better understand and keep in touch with the borderland between their subjects and clinical work.[19]

The strong opinions stated by the authors cited above were not universally shared among the academic leadership. W. H. Howell (professor of physiology at Johns Hopkins and holder of both M. D. and Ph.D. degrees) was most concerned that the teachers be "of the right sort." He was unsure of any difference between basic sciences taught as part of the university or "segregated with the clinical branches"; gains and losses existed with either model.

The medical student probably values more highly the medical surroundings. On the other hand, they have the disadvantage of distracting and diverting some students from a thorough study of the preparatory sciences. Some of our medical students chafe under this prolonged preparation, forgetting also that it gives them the badge, the impress that will differentiate them from the mere empiric, when the time comes for them to compete with their fellow practitioners.[20]

In summary, the 1910 basic science curriculum was characterized by marked differences among "good" and "poor" schools ("good" meaning institutions that had adopted the curricular reforms of the day). The modes of instruction, the qualifications of the faculty, and the facilities all were relevant to the quality of education that students received. Flexner's admonition that specifying curriculum structure would do no good, and could do harm, was largely unheeded. Both the AMA Council on Medical Education and the AAMC sponsored efforts to create a "model" curriculum, as a way to give direction and guidance to reform efforts.

THE BASIC SCIENCE CURRICULUM IN 1925

If in 1910 the "war" for curricular reform in the basic sciences still was being waged, by 1925 it had been won and the consequences of the "victory" were beginning to be recognized. Although there were half the number of medical schools in 1925 that there were in 1900,[21] the survivors had a number of problems. A national commission to study medical education reported that the

chief criticisms of the training in the medical sciences are directed against the presentation too early of too many details, often of temporary, miscellaneous, and inconsequential value, the overemphasis on the technical procedures of laboratory work, and the artificial segregation of the subjects.[22]

There still were differences among schools in the number of hours devoted to the basic sciences. In a 1925 survey of 66 medical schools, anatomy ranged from 432 to 1,185 hours, biological chemistry from 140 to 320 hours, physiology from 154 to 704 hours, pharmacology from 72 to 399 hours, and pathology/bacteriology from 304 to 830 hours, not a major change from 1910.[23]

The attempt to "provide instruction in too many subjects in too great detail" had "created great overcrowding of the curriculum." This was true across the basic sciences. The 1925 survey showed that about two-thirds of schools exceeded the AAMC-recommended number of hours in the basic science subjects: 43 exceeded the recommended number of hours in anatomy, 44 in pharmacology, 56 in physiology, 43 in biological chemistry, and 38 in pathology.[24]

Along with crowding, rigidity of the curriculum was being cited as a problem. Flexner, always an exponent of educational flexibility and freedom, wrote in 1925 that the desire to

stamp out unfit medical schools has also operated to strengthen regimentation ... our present fetters were therefore forged in order to compel wretched medical schools to give unfit medical students a 'better' training. Now that this end has been measurably accomplished, the means have become a fetish, blocking further improvement.[25]

The isolation of the basic sciences from the clinical disciplines, and from each other, was also being deplored. Basic science subjects were "more or less self-contained" and embraced a "wide range of specialized knowledge and technical methods." In many schools the student was "overwhelmed with the details and facts required," and success depended upon memory. The concentration plan of teaching was being blamed for the undesirable separation of the basic sciences from their clinical

applications. The chair of the AAMC's Committee on Curriculum acknowledged the fundamental importance of the basic sciences but
stressed that their "relation to the practice of medicine should at all times
be kept before the student."[26]

On the other side of this argument, there were representatives of the
basic sciences who felt that their disciplines were being subordinated to
practical applications. The results of a survey of physiologists and pharma-
cologists revealed the opinion that an emphasis on the "practical would be
detrimental" and that "major activities should be concentrated on fundamentals."[27]

The emphasis on laboratory teaching which had been central to curriculum reform also was being questioned. In the 1920s, students spent
considerable time in the laboratory. For example, surveys showed that
about 59 percent of course time in physiology and 76 percent of course
time in bacteriology were devoted to laboratory exercises. The concern
was raised in the *Final Report of the Commission on Medical Education* that
laboratory teaching had become an end in itself, and that the quality of
education was being judged by the amount of laboratory work. Too
much time was being spent in "unimportant and uninforming routine
experiments." What was really needed was the "cultivation of proper
intellectual attitude, which is not restricted to a single method of study."[28]

What were the reasons given for the curricular isolation of the basic
sciences and the emphasis on the content of the discipline, rather than
on its application to the practice of medicine? Many blamed the teachers,
who were felt to use their own special interests as the basis for selecting
what should be taught. Arthur Dean Bevan, still chair of the AMA
Council on Medical Education, complained in 1920 that many teachers
in the laboratory branches had drifted away from the science and practice
of medicine and from the medical profession. He reiterated that "men
of the non-medical type" had no place teaching the basic sciences.[29]

The 1925 standards of the Council on Medical Education echoed this
sentiment. They stated that there should be at least eight "expert, thoroughly trained professors in the laboratory branches," who should be
salaried so that they could devote full time to teaching and research.
These individuals should be graduates of medical schools and have training in all departments of medicine. "Non-medical men" should be employed as teachers only in "exceptional circumstances," where "medical
men of equal capacity" were not available.[30]

In reality, however, academic leaders already had recognized the difficulty of staffing the basic sciences with physicians. In 1920, the report
of a committee of the Division of Medical Sciences of the National Research Council was released. The committee was charged with studying
the availability of assistants in basic science departments. Ideally, the
assistant was a medical graduate doing research and teaching, prior to

taking a professorial position. The report stated that there was a shortage of satisfactory assistants, that the "better graduates" did not join the basic science departments, and if they did join, did not stay long. One major reason cited was insufficient salaries, and the disparity in incomes between basic science and clinical faculty members. Problems recruiting physicians for the basic sciences were balanced by the increased availability of individuals with Ph.D. degrees. The better departments were offering graduate programs to train their own future faculty members.[31]

Various solutions were implemented for the curricular problems of the 1920s. One approach by the AAMC was to develop a model curriculum which allotted each subject a percent of the total instead of a specific number of hours. For example, anatomy should occupy 14 to 18.5 percent of the total and physiology 4.5 to 6 percent. It was believed that this would facilitate curricular flexibility. Another, more direct, strategy was for medical schools to reduce the total number of instructional hours. For example, a sample of 13 schools showed that the total number of hours decreased from an average of 4,378 in 1925 to 3,914 in 1928.[32]

THE BASIC SCIENCE CURRICULUM IN 1940

In 1940, concern was being raised about the range in quality among the 77 medical schools and about the tendency in some schools to admit more students than the laboratory and hospital facilities could accommodate.[33] A national survey of medical education, planned by the AMA Council on Medical Education, the AAMC, and the Federation of State Medical Boards, was conducted between 1934 and 1939. The survey evaluated medical school departments in terms of their personnel, physical facilities, financial support, educational programs, and research efforts. The departments that were rated highest followed the Flexner model: they had sufficient space and suitable facilities, a good faculty-student ratio, emphasized laboratory teaching with an experimental point of view, and had ongoing research programs with graduate biomedical education components.[34]

There was still a "block" system in the basic science curriculum; the trend was for students to complete anatomy, biochemistry, and physiology in the first year and pathology, bacteriology, and pharmacology in the second year. In some schools, however, bacteriology was taught in the first year and in others physiology extended into the second year. Physical diagnosis and brief courses in clinical subjects also appeared in the second year. In the four year schools, gross anatomy ranged from 220 to 600 hours, biochemistry from 100 to 360 hours, physiology from 180 to 556 hours, pharmacology from 88 to 273 hours, bacteriology from 90 to 326 hours, and pathology from 176 to 396 hours. While there still was a range in the numbers of hours, there was a downward shift from previous periods. Laboratory occupied about 62 percent of total basic science hours.[35]

In what were rated as the poorer schools in the national survey, the curriculum was felt to be "merely a mimicry of nonmedical university courses practically devoid of any medical and clinical implications." Frog physiology had been deplored by many since the 1920s. The use of lower animals in the laboratory was being replaced by the use of mammalian and human experiments, especially in what were characterized as the "better schools." Teachers in these institutions taught the principles of the basic medical sciences using human examples and laboratory experiments relevant to clinical medicine.[36]

What factors influenced curriculum content in 1940? The discipline-based, as opposed to the practice-based, perspective still acted as a determinant of curriculum content. The content of licensing board examinations was raised as another factor that affected what instructors taught. Whatever the feelings of teachers, "every medical student must learn to juggle enough details" to pass these examinations. Boards "set up objectives, which, like taxes, cannot well be evaded." The author of this sentiment analyzed and categorized the content of anatomy questions given by ten examining boards in tests between 1932 and 1938. He found that of 1,005 questions, about 42 percent were requests for descriptions or definitions and 37 percent asked for direct information, lists, or outlines. Thus, a total of about three-quarters of the questions covered detail that did not require high levels of analysis or synthesis.[37]

Concern about the increased number of students led to an evaluation of the number and competence of faculty members. Total faculty:student ratios (including faculty members of all ranks from professor to fellow-assistant) ranged from 1:2 to 1:12 across medical schools (median 1:5.3). In 1936, there were 2,594 basic science faculty members, with 42 percent holding the rank of assistant professor or above. Of the total number of basic science faculty members, 22 percent held only the Ph.D. degree, 55 percent held the M.D. degree, and 23 percent held no degree or a degree other than the M.D. or Ph.D. In 66 four-year medical schools, the following percentages of department chairs held the M.D. degree: anatomy, 70 percent; biochemistry, 26 percent; physiology, 64 percent; microbiology, 74 percent; pathology, 98 percent; and pharmacology, 83 percent. Thus, by the late 1930s, it was usual for nonphysicians to be department chairs in some of the basic sciences.[38]

By 1940, leaders in medical education had concluded that it was impossible to teach medical students all they needed to know. The objective of medical education, at least in the better schools, was to give students a "sound foundation."[39] Adhering to this principle would allow inclusion of appropriate content and prevent further overcrowding. However, there was no general consensus about what, in the basic sciences, should be included in this foundation. This uncertainty continued into the next period, as the existing problems became intensified.

THE BASIC SCIENCE CURRICULUM IN 1955

In general, this was a time of re-examination, without, however, widely-accepted proposals for significant change. A national survey of medical education, sponsored by the Association of American Medical Colleges, included visits to forty-one of the eighty-one medical schools[40] and collection of questionnaire data from all schools. In addition, the association sponsored a number of "Teaching Institutes" in the mid–1950s. These brought together medical school faculty members and administrators to discuss the current status of medical education and to make recommendations for change.[41]

The general curriculum structure was relatively consistent across schools and the amount of time devoted to individual subjects was generally similar to that in 1940. By this time, it was common for the basic sciences to share the first two years of the curriculum with other subjects. The increasing amount of content, resulting from the addition of new information, contributed to the lengthening of the school year and to excessive amounts of didactic teaching in some subjects. The first year contained an average of 1,000 to 1,200 hours. Of these, anatomy (including gross anatomy, neuroanatomy, microanatomy, and embryology) ranged from 770 to 408 hours (median about 600), biochemistry ranged from 338 to 144 hours (median about 230), and physiology ranged from 440 to 100 hours (median about 165). Many schools also gave short didactic courses in statistics, public health, medical history, and medical physics. Correlation clinics, which involved faculty members from clinical departments, commonly were held once per week. Psychology/psychiatry, covering normal personality development and psychobiology, was taught in about two-thirds of schools.

In the second year, the student could be exposed to as many as 8 to 15 separate courses, but the majority of time still was devoted to basic science subjects. Pharmacology ranged from 358 to 80 hours (median 165), microbiology ranged from 327 to 144 hours (median 224), and pathology ranged from 462 to 108 hours (median 312). The second part of the year was considered a transition to the clinical disciplines. Clinical departments often gave lectures or short introductory courses. Consequently, there was little free time in the curriculum. The norm was for students to be free one weekday afternoon and Saturday afternoon. In both first- and second-year basic science subjects, except for pharmacology, laboratory occupied an average of at least one-half the scheduled hours.[42]

A perception had existed to some degree for at least thirty years that the curriculum was overcrowded and fragmented. To address these problems, one theme that emerged from several of the AAMC teaching institutes was the desire to enhance curricular integration among the basic sciences and between basic science and clinical disciplines.

In the early 1950s, a new model of basic science instruction was introduced that had curricular integration as one of its foundations. This was Western Reserve (later Case-Western Reserve) University's move to an organ-systems-based curriculum in 1952. Instead of discipline-based courses, content was organized by body system (for example, cardiovascular, gastrointestinal). The Western Reserve model was developed in response to problems with the existing curriculum, including competition among departments for teaching time, a lack of correlation of content among the departments, and a lack of agreement about what a graduate of the school should know and be able to do. The curriculum was designed to integrate basic science teaching across disciplines and to heighten the relevance of the basic sciences to clinical medicine. The broad objectives of the medical program stressed the correlation of teaching concerning human biology, the principles of medicine, and care of the patient. This curriculum innovation was facilitated by an organizational change: the faculty as a whole, through its committee structure rather than individual departments, was vested with responsibility for the curriculum. The Western Reserve "experiment" was a model for many curriculum change efforts in the 1960s and 1970s.[43]

The number of basic science faculty members was increasing, but not in proportion to the increase in the number of students. In addition to their medical school teaching responsibilities, medical school faculty taught students working for advanced degrees in the basic sciences, as well as public health, dental, and nursing students. This increasing teaching commitment led to concerns about a future faculty shortage. The importance of training degree candidates in the basic sciences, in both medical schools and universities, was recognized, and the important role of non-physicians in medical education was acknowledged by organizations such as the AAMC. In some basic science departments, the percent of non-physician faculty members was increasing. The proportion of faculty members with M.D. degrees ranged from less than 20 percent in biochemistry departments to greater than 95 percent in pathology departments.[44]

The 1950s was a period of relative calm in medical education. The Western Reserve "experiment" received attention, but widespread initiatives for change were lacking. This is in contrast to the significant activity of the next two decades.

THE BASIC SCIENCE CURRICULUM IN 1970

Starting in about the mid–1960s, a number of new medical schools were founded and the class size of existing schools increased. This occurred in response to a perceived shortage of physicians in the United States. During the 1970–71 academic year, there were 103 medical schools, 97 with four-year programs and 6 with two-year programs. This represents more than a 20 percent increase from 1955. The number of accepted applicants to medical school increased from 7,969 in 1955–56 to 11,500 in 1970–71.[45]

The growth stimulated curricular change. A survey of medical schools in 1970–71 showed that 90 percent of established schools had made major curricular changes in the past five years or were planning a curricular revision at the time. Many of the changes involved a blurring of the traditional division of the curriculum into two years of basic science and two clinical years. Attempts were made to identify a core curriculum in the basic sciences, to reduce repetition and to eliminate less relevant information. The curricular changes were not, however, universally accepted. One basic science faculty member attributed the changes to the desire of the clinical departments to diminish the role of basic scientists in medical education.[46]

There was a trend toward curricular integration in the basic sciences. In 1972–73, twenty-one schools had an integrated curriculum, most commonly with an organ-systems type of organization, instead of individual courses. Many other schools introduced one or more interdepartmental courses, such as neurosciences or cell biology.[47]

For the schools that retained a discipline-based format, the average number of hours in anatomy (including gross anatomy, histology, embryology, and neuroanatomy) was 332, in biochemistry 141, in physiology 161, in microbiology 140, in pathology 243, and in pharmacology 123. These represent a significant decrease as compared to 1955, in part a result of a reduction or elimination of laboratory hours. The total curricular time in the first two years remained about constant. New basic science courses (such as genetics, cell biology, pathophysiology), early clinical experiences, and behavioral science/psychiatry courses were added to replace the lost basic science hours.[48]

Associated with expansion of medical education was an increase in the number of basic science faculty members. In addition, as compared with 1940, the percentage of department heads with M.D. degrees had decreased in all basic sciences but pathology.[49]

The dynamic curricular changes of the decade were tied to a period of expansion. In the next period, growth began to slow and many of the innovations of the 1960s and 1970s came under review.

THE BASIC SCIENCE CURRICULUM IN 1985 AND BEYOND

The 1980s were characterized by re-examination of the curriculum. Major studies were sponsored by the AMA Council on Medical Education

and the Association of American Medical Colleges, and the reports highlighted a number of problems with the current system. In general, it
was felt that the environment of medicine was changing and that medical
education was not adapting rapidly enough.[50]

Many of the innovations introduced in the previous period had been
abandoned by the mid–1980s. For example, more than one-half of the
schools with a predominantly organ-systems-based basic science curriculum in 1973 had a discipline-based curriculum by 1984. However, a
new approach to curricular integration emerged in the 1970s and 1980s:
problem-based learning. In this format, the basic sciences are organized
according to their relevance in addressing defined clinical problems (for
example, an individual presenting with chest pain, an infant with failure
to thrive). This model has been advocated as a means to ensure the
relevance of basic science content to eventual practice and a way to
facilitate retention of information acquired during the first two years.
While only two of the 126 U.S. medical schools employ problem-based
learning as the major curricular format, six others have a problem-based
track, and ninety-six offer some problem-based learning experiences in
one or more courses.[51]

The number of basic science hours has continued to decrease. There
were an average of 1,734 total hours in years one and two of the curriculum. Of these, 1,286 (74 percent) were occupied by the traditional
six basic sciences. The average number of hours devoted to anatomy
was 297, to biochemistry 120, to physiology 142, to microbiology 120,
to pathology 162, and to pharmacology 111—all below the averages in
the early 1970s. Of basic science hours, 29 percent was devoted to the
laboratory, as compared to 62 percent in 1940. Behavioral science and
related subjects occupied about 5 percent of total hours in the first two
years.[52]

The number of basic science faculty members has increased, even
though the number of medical schools and class sizes have been relatively
stable since the early 1980s. Except for pathology, the trend toward non-
physicians as department heads continued. In 1984, 27 percent of anatomy department heads, 13 percent of biochemistry department heads,
35 percent of physiology department heads, 35 percent of microbiology
department heads, 51 percent of pharmacology department heads, and
98 percent of pathology department heads held the M.D. degree.[53]

CONCLUSIONS

It is clear that both stability and change characterize the preclinical
portion of the medical curriculum during the twentieth century. The
amount of time devoted to the basic sciences has decreased, the emphasis
on laboratory teaching has declined, and new subjects areas have been

incorporated. However, the relative placement of the basic science subjects has remained stable, and the discipline-based, concentration plan
of curriculum organization is again dominant. The themes elaborated
at the beginning of the chapter—the relationship of the basic sciences
to the clinical disciplines, the training of faculty members, the means to
prevent curriculum overcrowding—serve as a summary of the controversies of the past eighty years.

The dispute over how much practical orientation the basic sciences
should be given still exists. The issue continues to divide instructors along
disciplinary lines, with clinical faculty members favoring an applied focus
for content selection and basic science faculty members advocating a
discipline-oriented approach. Since the decision about what to teach is
usually left to individual departments, the discipline-based focus pre-
dominates. Problem-based learning is an exception, in that basic science
content is tied to specific clinical situations. In integrated curriculum
formats with an applied orientation (organ-systems- or problem-based
learning), success requires an organizational structure that permits non-
departmental input into the selection of content—for example, a curriculum committee charged with broad authority for making curricular
decisions.[54]

The difference in educational background between faculty members
and administrators in basic science departments and in clinical departments has been widening throughout the century. While leaders in medical education first protested the employment of non-physicians, this
soon became an acknowledged fact of life. For at least the last forty
years, holders of Ph.D. degrees have been the majority of faculty members in most basic science departments. In addition, the need to increase
the number of basic science faculty members led to the recruitment of
many instructors who obtained their training in university, as opposed
to medical school, departments. This has enhanced the separation of
the two camps within the medical school.

Throughout the twentieth century commentators have expressed concern that the basic science curriculum was overcrowded. Why did this
perennial perception exist? One element was the large amount of time
that students spent in the classroom or laboratory. Through mid-century,
unscheduled time was rare and elective time infrequent. Students were
expected to learn through didactic experiences, not through independent study or self-selected activities. Another cause was the frequent
addition of new subject areas, often incorporated as short courses requiring examination time. Even if the absolute number of hours did not
increase, the addition of examinations created more pressure for students. It also is probable that while the traditional basic sciences lost
scheduled hours, they did not correspondingly decrease the amount of
content that was covered. This hypothesis is supported by the increasing

amount of time spent on didactic, as opposed to laboratory, teaching as the century progressed. Again, departmentally-based decisions about what and how much to include were the guiding force behind curriculum, once the overall number of hours was assigned to a given course. The concept of a "core curriculum," that would make explicit what all students should learn, was never generally accepted.

What would Abraham Flexner think of the basic science curriculum today? He would probably applaud the excellent training of current faculty members, and regret that many appear to be indifferent to teaching. He would approve of current efforts to implement active learning experiences, such as problem-based learning, and would criticize the loss of laboratory time. The relative lack of flexibility in the curriculum also would disappoint him. He would suggest that students be given more freedom to learn the basic sciences in multiple ways, that didactic lectures be minimized, and that the long hours that many students spend in class be reduced. In general, he would say what others attempting to reform medical education today are saying. With all the change that has occurred throughout the century, it is ironic that the problems with basic science education, and the ways to proposed to solve them, have changed least of all.

3

Clinical Education Since Flexner or Whatever Became of William Osler?

Edward C. Atwater

Commencement at Johns Hopkins Medical School in 1905 marked the departure of two people, one a student and one a professor, who were symbolic of the changes that were to come to clinical education in the decades ahead, especially the diminishing influence of the practitioner. Graduating that day and about to start his career was George Hoyt Whipple. In sixteen years he would become the founding dean of the University of Rochester Medical School, the first new school after Abraham Flexner's scathing 1910 report.[1] That institution owed its existence in large part to Flexner's effort to universalize the clinical full-time system by outflanking the recalcitrant New York City schools with a new school upstate.[2] Also, the fact that Whipple was a pathologist reflected the growing trend to appointment of non-clinicians as deans. Before this time, most schools had been led by practitioners. By 1921, more than a quarter of the nation's eighty medical schools had "laboratory men" as deans.[3]

As Whipple began his career, one of his professors, William Osler, first professor of medicine at Johns Hopkins, was retiring to become Regius Professor at Oxford. Osler was fifty-six and the exemplary generalist consultant of his day. He was, however, overwhelmed by the demands of those who sought his professional counsel and felt that he was "on the downgrade." He had vowed to "chuck everything" at sixty, in any case.[4] The offer from England was his golden parachute.

The year 1905 was also important in less symbolic ways. The number of American medical schools reached a high of 160. A subsequent decrease in the number of schools and, more importantly, in the number of students, and a sharp increase in the per-student income of schools made it possible to require better educational preparation of students, to establish the clinical clerkship as the basic method of undergraduate instruction, and to provide salaries for clinical faculty.[5]

The departure of Osler and the graduation of Whipple were portents of the decline of the clinician and the ascendancy of the laboratory man, as well as the appearance of the professional medical educator, in American medical education. No one was more aware of this changing balance than Osler himself: leaving the commencement platform that day, he turned to his colleague, Professor of Anatomy Franklin P. Mall, and remarked, "Now I go and you have your way."[6] The "way" was to establish full-time chairs at Johns Hopkins that would provide adequate salaries for professors of medicine, surgery, and pediatrics. These professors would then cease to be dependent on practice income and could devote their entire time to teaching and research, just as the professors of biochemistry, bacteriology, and pathology did.

Though the burden of practice played a major role in Osler's decision to leave Johns Hopkins, he also thought that the full-time plan was inherently flawed. To some, being a physician was like playing the violin, a performing art that required daily practice. Osler was concerned lest professors become a "set of clinical prigs" and he feared that "the broad open spirit which has characterized the school should narrow, as teacher and student chased each other down the fascinating road of research, forgetful of those wider interests to which a great hospital must minister."[7]

Though Osler's prediction turned out to be an accurate one, there was, nevertheless, another side to the matter. The reformers correctly perceived serious flaws in the educational system as it then existed. There were too many doctors being graduated. There was no minimum standard of intelligence required to matriculate at an American medical school, and many of those who attended could barely read and write. A large number, probably most, of the students were not prepared for the laboratory work that was becoming part of medicine. Since most medical schools provided little or no laboratory training, this deficiency often went unexposed and uncorrected. Most clinical faculties were composed of local practitioners who themselves knew little of laboratory methods or research, and for whom teaching was a part-time activity. By reducing the number of schools and the number of students at each school, and by establishing a corps of salaried full-time clinicians who would emphasize teaching and research, Flexner and his supporters hoped to correct these problems. If there were fears that a fundamental temperamental disparity existed between those who find satisfaction in practice and those who love the quest for new knowledge, two kinds of work in which the interpersonal relationships and the reward systems are so very different, these fears were suppressed. It was assumed that the investigator could teach students about practice.

Figure 3.1
American Medical Education, 1900–1930

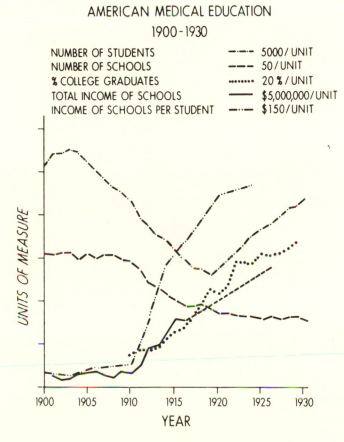

AMERICAN MEDICAL EDUCATION
1900-1930

NUMBER OF STUDENTS	—·—·— 5000/UNIT
NUMBER OF SCHOOLS	— — — 50/UNIT
% COLLEGE GRADUATES	········ 20 %/UNIT
TOTAL INCOME OF SCHOOLS	——— $5,000,000/UNIT
INCOME OF SCHOOLS PER STUDENT	—··—··— $150/UNIT

Source: From E. C. Atwater, "Financial Subsidies for American Medical Education Before 1940." Master's Essay, Johns Hopkins University Baltimore, 1974.

The proposed changes did, in fact, come. In part they were the results of forces already in motion when Flexner appeared on the scene. Flexner, and the financial backers he represented, played an important role in accomplishing changes that had long been sought. Between 1910 and 1925 the number of medical schools decreased by almost 50 percent, and the number of medical students, already down from a peak of 27,000 in 1904, fell as low as 14,000 by the end of World War I before starting gradually upward again. The annual per-student income of schools rose from $75 to $700 (Figure 3.1). In 1906 only five of 162 schools required two years of college preparation, but by 1918 eighty of eighty-nine did (Figure 3.2). At last it became possible to hire full-time clinical faculty, give individual bedside instruction, provide clinical laboratories, and

Figure 3.2
Premedical Requirements

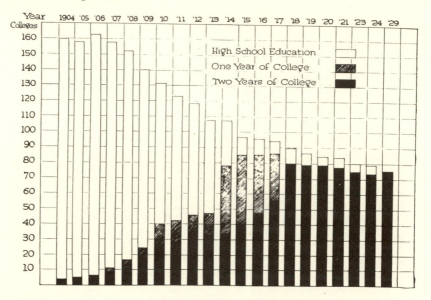

Source: "Medical Education in the United States," *Journal of the American Medical Association* 95 (1930): 507.

have students who were able to comprehend what they were doing. By 1925, the clinical clerkship, an experience that offered each student bedside experience and responsibility, was universal in American medical schools, and schools were establishing effective control over or at least developing a working relationship with the hospitals they used for clinical teaching.

MAJOR CHANGES IN MEDICINE SINCE 1910

Four major changes in medicine have affected clinical teaching since 1910. The first was the establishment of university control over hospitals and clinical faculties and the replacement of the practitioner by the full-time academic clinical investigator as role model for students. Equally important was the steady expansion of more sophisticated technology which, later propelled by prosperity, promoted specialism. A third element was the passing of financial control from individuals and philanthropists to third parties and bureaus, whether prepaid insurers, government welfare programs, or federal training and research subsidies. Perhaps most important of all was a period of unusual prosperity and an increased expectation and willingness on the part of the public to spend money in pursuit of its own health and longevity. These changes influenced the structure of clinical training and also affected the type of person who chose medicine as a profession.

By the end of the nineteenth century, it had become customary for a school to accept as professor of a clinical discipline that person who had risen through the ranks of the local profession to be chief of service at the hospital. Such a person was primarily in private practice. As the chief of a hospital service, he controlled the beds needed for clinical instruction of clerks and house officers. Therefore, if schools were to select their clinical professors from a national pool and not simply appoint the senior physicians from the local hospital staffs, they would need to control hospitals. Such necessity was the driving force behind the Johns Hopkins Hospital, the Peter Bent Brigham Hospital, and Strong Memorial Hospital, among others.

Nowhere was the transition to recruiting faculty from a national pool more striking than at Harvard. In 1890, the entire senior medical faculty was Boston-born and -trained, and largely interconnected by marriage. After 1892, an increasing number of "outsiders" joined the pre-clinical faculty. In 1908, the first non-Bostonian clinician, Henry A. Christian, came from Johns Hopkins as professor of medicine. He had to be installed at a minor hospital until the Brigham was completed. The coup de grace was the importation in 1912 of David Edsall as physician-in-chief at the Massachusetts General Hospital, an appointment which by-passed Boston's heir-apparent for the position, Richard C. Cabot. By 1920, only two senior Boston-born physicians held major clinical posts at Harvard.[8]

This type of change occurred in other places, too. Soon, the medical schools controlled the major hospitals, and the faculty had been nationalized and put on salary. This cohort of salaried clinicians gave momentum to the development of laboratory medicine, new technology, and ever greater specialization.

As the technology of medicine increased in complexity, the status of the senior generalist consultant was further eroded. In the early part of the twentieth century the state of medical art was predominantly that of bedside physical diagnosis, which had evolved during the preceding century.[9] The use of the x-ray was hardly common, and laboratory medicine was in its infancy. The great advances that characterized research prior to 1960 were accomplished largely in the clinical laboratory: assaying cellular, molecular, ionic, electrical, hormonal, and antibody elements and developing vaccines, replacement hormones and fluids, and antibiotics. The scope of these innovations, however, remained within the comprehension of any physician who chose to attain competence. This was soon to change.

The trend toward specialism was further accelerated in the years of post-World War II prosperity and subsidies for research. The devel-

opments of many effective pharmacological agents, chemical manipulation of body fluids, improved anesthesia, assisted ventilation, extra-
corporeal cardiovascular support, blood ("renal") dialysis, reconstructive
and transplantation surgery, microsurgery, and the application of the
computer to radiology greatly increased diagnostic and therapeutic ver-
satility, as well as the costs of health care. As medicine became dependent
on complex technology, what had to be learned during training changed.
Unlike the classical physical examination, the ward laboratory, and even
the early radiographic machines, the new technology could not be employed by each individual physician. Physicians gradually lost self-suf-
ficiency, and some of the feeling of personal, individual responsibility
for patients. This altered the type of person who found medicine an
appealing profession.

Another element that affected clinical education was the development
of third-party payment for hospital care. Having started in the mid–
1930s, the "Blue Plans" were greatly extended after World War II when
industrial labor sought coverage as a benefit and management considered this good business policy. Since most third-party insurers paid the
hospital the calculated per diem cost, there was little incentive to be
economical. The price of hospital care soared, especially after 1965 when
Medicare was established. The strong preference of the reward system
for technical procedures rather than verbal and physical communication
changed the character of practice by encouraging the use of tests and
discouraging listening and thinking.

Also, with increasingly reliable sources of income, hospitals ceased to
be eleemosynary institutions. They were soon to be run on business
principles by professional administrators. Lawsuits became more frequent and were more often successful. The character of medical practice
and teaching changed in keeping with these changes. The role of the
physician, whether as student, resident, or attending, became less pa-
ternalistic and more adversarial after money came to medicine.

Not only was there interposition of a bureaucracy controlling the purse
of "paying patients," those who had a steady source of income, but a
welfare system operated by public employees also was created, to assume
administrative responsibility for the poor. This was probably a necessary
and inevitable innovation, but it changed medical practice and clinical
teaching by altering the transaction between patient and physician. On
an individual level, free care of the poor by private arrangement between
patient and physician had, since Hippocratic times, given the physician
a sense of social responsibility and personal commitment. This fundamental obligation diminished and, with that, something changed in the
natural selection of matriculants for medicine. At an institutional level,
the disappearance of the non-paying or ward patient greatly altered the
process of clinical education. Though intended to equalize the social

aspects of hospital care by giving all patients senior attending physicians, in reality the change often merely transferred the responsibility to a senior physician without engendering the interest that the younger physicians-in-training had previously shown. It is not clear that the so-called welfare or Medicaid patient receives better or even as good care under the present socially more egalitarian and more costly system. Also, the decline in responsibility given to physicians-in-training may have deleterious effects on their development.

Most significant of all the changes was the rather rapid transition from a resignation, a submission to the frailties and evils of life and the hopeful belief in a better life hereafter, to a conviction that science and prosperity could solve all problems (if sufficiently supported). Attention turned increasingly from the life to come to the life here on earth.

CHANGES IN CLINICAL EDUCATION

What changes have actually occurred in clinical education since 1905 as a result of the four elements just described? In an effort to establish an orderly arrangement of many complex, interrelated themes, I have chosen to look at the effects these four elements had in five different areas: the site of teaching, primarily the hospital; the body of knowledge to be addressed, or the curriculum; the patients; the teachers; and the students.

The Hospital

The hospital gradually changed from a relatively intimate domestic household dependent on gifts and donations for its survival to a distribution center for "high technology" that is run on business principles. It ceased to be a place where the patient came for comfort and nursing while awaiting the outcome of an illness and became a place where patients sought highly specific services. No longer eleemosynary, it became subject to the legal doctrine of *respondeat superior*, which holds the employer responsible for the acts of employees performed in the line of duty. American hospitals had long been exempted from this liability for fear that their precarious existence would be jeopardized. With the passing of this vulnerability, lawsuits became more frequent and successful, changing the character of hospital practice and teaching, making the institution more efficient and careful, but also less comforting.

The hospital today has an atmosphere entirely different from that of even forty years ago. The teaching function, though still important, is less obvious among its many other expanded activities. Though the hospital is still central to clinical education, the reasons for this centrality have changed. Fifty years ago the hospital provided a setting in which patients could be examined periodically during the course of an illness, both directly and by means of the laboratory available nearby. Today, the hospital has become so enormous, so complex that this simplest teaching function is dwarfed. The image of the hospital has improved from that of a place to be avoided to one where wrong is made right. It has in many ways replaced the church as the institution to which most turn for help in time of trouble. The increasing technological function of the hospital, however, makes it a less satisfactory setting than it used to be for students and for patient-centered learning.

The Curriculum

The changes in knowledge and curriculum are no less striking. A survey done by D. J. DeSolla Price in 1963 concluded that the world's scientific literature increased exponentially after 1750, doubling every fifteen years.[10] While this does not quite prove that we know twice as much every fifteen years, only perhaps that more people are "doing research" and publishing, the statistic does give some idea of the boundaries of information that each succeeding generation of young physicians must consider.

When William Beaumont did his studies of gastric secretion through a fistula to the stomach of his patient Alexis St. Martin in the 1820s and 1830s, clinical research in America was an exceptional activity. That Beaumont could perform his investigations depended on the fact that he was a salaried Army Medical Officer with the backing of his superior, the Surgeon-General. Half a century later the Philadelphia physician S. Weir Mitchell did significant clinical research in the evening, though he practiced all day and was still available to his patients at night. He supported his activities through his own efforts. When patrons appeared to sponsor clinical research, whether foundations or the government, and it was no longer necessary to pay for one's own time, a cadre of professional investigators soon appeared. Combined with this new mode of financing was a rapidly evolving technology, stimulated by war and prosperity. The result was an enormous increase in real knowledge and an even larger expansion of information.[11]

Since one cannot encompass the whole field of clinical medicine in the years of formal schooling, it seemed reasonable to identify a manageable body of essential information to be learned and, at the same time, to concentrate on teaching a method that could be applied to unfamiliar situations. The method that evolved was that of individual case study and the setting in which it was used was the clinical clerkship. The virtue of the case study method was that it focused all the information, historical, physical, and laboratory, some of which would turn out to be important and some of which would be less important, on a particular patient and a particular problem. Hence, the student was not dealing with vast amounts of data in the abstract.[12]

Other ways to cope with this information explosion have included attempts to define a core curriculum and to introduce more electives. The attempt after mid-century to identify a core curriculum assumed that it was more important for students to have learned about congestive heart failure and to have cared for a patient with this problem than it was for them to have been exposed to some esoteric entity: students should think of zebras when they hear hoofbeats, but they should think of horses first. Another attempt to deal with the information explosion was the establishment of clinical electives. These allowed students to concentrate on areas in which they were more interested or to which they wanted some exposure prior to pursuing an alternative clinical specialty. Electives were practical from the school's point of view because so many faculty were now specialty-focused.

The content of the curriculum gradually changed, as did the types of problems seen in the hospital. To the generation trained in the 1920s and 1930s, pneumonia, syphilis, tuberculosis, congestive heart failure, strokes, abdominal and gynecological surgery, fractures, and pediatric infectious disease with its related complications were the most common problems. By 1990, the picture was quite different, with infectious disease less common, surgery applied regularly and far more boldly to all parts of the body, and a marked increase in the chronic neurological, neoplastic, and degenerative problems seen in older populations. Most important from the pedagogical point of view, the diagnostic procedures, the care, and the treatment all became more complicated and risky.

One victim of the "Germano-Flexner" emphasis on science, at both premedical and clinical levels, was the broader base of humanistic learning. The balance shifted toward excellence in science, which had made possible the spectacular advances in medicine, and away from a competent use of English and a knowledge of the historical continuum in which medicine operates. Today, there is a double curricular standard in medical schools, strict in the scientific part of medicine but more casual in the humanities. A pre-medical student is required to do well in organic chemistry but may fulfill the English language requirement with no more than a passing grade in "advertising English." Instead of rigorous electives in English, history, or philosophy, humanities courses in medical schools can consist of "bull" sessions in ethics, "store-front" economics, and no composition training at all. Despite talk of the need for broad education of physicians, time and cost constraints today impose the same impregnable barrier in the humanities that prevented reform of the science curriculum in proprietary schools in 1900. If undergraduate students preparing for medicine hear the admonition to seek broad intellectual experience, they put it in the context of "do as I say, not as I do."

The Patients

The population of patients in hospitals has changed considerably since 1905. This is due to various factors: the changing spectrum of disease, especially infectious disease, with the constant change in pathogenicity of microorganisms (such as streptococcus); the coming of antibiotics; the imposition of public health measures; and especially the development of effective vaccines. But it is the ability of the hospital to function as a "high-tech" depot instead of a nursing infirmary that has been mainly responsible for the difference in patients. The larger teaching hospitals admit patients with a narrower range of problems than formerly. The patients are sicker, often too sick for beginning students to care for. Also patients stay in the hospital too short a time and are often away from the ward for tests and treatments. They must be shared with a growing number of graduates-in-training. Surgical patients have an increasing number of procedures done outside the hospital and often have brief hospital stays. More and more of the diagnostic workup in medicine and surgery is done before admission. Due to these changes, the hospitalized patient now illustrates the natural history of disease even less well than before and is therefore less satisfactory for teaching.

Nor are patients anymore the passive recipients of an omniscient physician's ministrations; they are consumers served by providers. They have rights. They give informed consent. They participate in decisions regarding all aspects of their care and treatment. The disappearance of the ward or charity patient, especially after 1965, broadened the patient population by making private patients available for teaching for the first time, but residents, especially in surgery, now have less responsibility for their patients than under the old system.

The Clinical Teachers

The teachers, too, have changed. As specialism has developed, the generalist has found it increasingly difficult to conduct bedside rounds. Lawrence Kohn, who was chief resident in medicine at Strong Memorial Hospital when it opened in 1925, and who practiced in Rochester for forty-six years, was a strong defender of the practitioner-teacher. In 1953 he wrote, "since we have begun to teach the theory of observing and treating the whole man, it is the medical man with some years of experience who would appear best able to show this theory in action." He thought it "unreasonable to expect a practitioner to expound on potassium or serum iron, but it is equally unlikely that a full-time instructor should understand gout as a disease."[13] The practitioner is better able to recognize the importance of personal problems in individuals reporting illness *before* all the tests come back negative.

In spite of Kohn's belief, between 1955 and 1975 the proportion of part-time faculty-practitioners who served as attending physicians on the medical wards of Strong Memorial Hospital fell from 50 percent to less than 15 percent.[14] Now even full-time faculty are finding it difficult to perform this task. Bedside teaching is done increasingly by those highly trained in subspecialty areas and selected in consideration of the problem presented by the patient. The generalist attending physician has become almost an anachronism. The role survives partly because of the need to preserve some comprehensive authority in both teaching and patient care. But as the cycle of fashion has swung toward the clinical faculty supporting itself by practice fees, the teacher-clinician is again restricted in the time he or she can devote to teaching and limited by ever-narrower experience.[15]

Perhaps the biggest change of all is in the status of the physician in the hospital. Once an authoritative, dominant figure in a charitable institution wholly dependent on his willingness to donate time in return for a sense of service or prestige, the physician is now part of a team, all of whose members work together. This has certain advantages as far as learning and quality control are concerned, but it makes day-to-day functioning more complicated. There is also an element of stress from the scrutiny of peer-review teams, third-party payers, lawyers, and governmental agencies. Teaching has inevitably come to play a smaller role in the attention of the hospital-based clinician.

The Student

And what of the student? Clinical teaching has clearly changed from a focus on undergraduate medical education to one on graduate medical education, that is to specialty training for residents and subspecialty training for fellows. This has followed ineluctably from the ever more demanding requirements for specialty certification, the ever greater desire of young physicians for specialty status, and the need of hospital-based specialists for junior assistants. This changing emphasis, combined with the changing characteristics of the hospitalized patient and the clinical teacher, is threatening the classical clinical clerkship.

By the 1920s, with more income and smaller classes in medical schools, the clerkship had become the standard method of undergraduate clinical instruction. Not a new idea, it traced its lineage at least to seventeenth-century Holland and came to the United States from Berlin via Dublin. Earlier attempts to establish it in America, notably at New Orleans, failed because the format required many teachers, many patients, few students, and hospitals that would tolerate what Lloyd Stevenson has called the responsible student. It was not until the organization of the Johns Hopkins School of Medicine that proper conditions existed for establishment of the clinical clerkship in the United States.[16]

The clinical clerk learned to deal with patients under the guidance of an instructor or preceptor. The clerk formed an ongoing relationship with the patient, took a history, did a complete physical examination, re-examined the patient from day to day and began to understand the meaning of changing physical signs. Thus, the clerk performed a service to the patient and to his or her primary teachers, the residents, by doing such tasks as bedside phlebotomies and laboratory procedures in the name of learning. In return, the student gained access to the patient and the attention of the resident.

Previously, clerks had defined responsibility. Now, clerks no longer have as significant a role in patient management. This is partly because the patient is less available, being often away having tests or treatments; partly because technicians have assumed many of the functions once filled by clerks; and partly because the hospital, now liable, fears greater risk from work done by less experienced personnel. Clerks do less than they once did in the way of nursing care. Their menial chores are no longer considered a learning experience now that third parties pay hospital personnel for such tasks. Tests are done in distant laboratories by technicians. Even the physical examination is becoming less important in a time of computers. The clerk's relationship with residents and patients is more passive, and the maturing element of responsibility is thereby diminished. The clerk, less useful to hospital, to teachers, and to patients, has been relegated to the conference room.

At the same time, increasing specialization has brought a need for more extended and focused graduate education. Toward the end of the nineteenth century, the internship, which consisted of a year or two of hospital service after the medical degree, was reserved for the most promising graduates. By the middle of the 1920s, it had become possible for all students to spend a postgraduate hospital year. For example, in 1925 there were 3,974 graduates of American medical schools and 3,832 internship positions; in 1930, there were 4,565 graduates and 5,531 internship positions.[17] An internship was also made a requirement, partly to remedy the deficient or almost absent undergraduate clinical experience that existed in American schools before the clinical clerkship was established, and partly because hospitals needed cheap ward physicians. The internship year included general clinical experiences that became gradually less essential as clerkships improved and residencies were extended.

The specialized graded residency, like the clerkship, evolved at Johns

Hopkins, where Halsted introduced the method being used by Billroth in Germany. Again, at first, the best and the brightest were selected for advanced training, and from among them only the most able survived. In thirty-three years Halsted had only seventeen chief residents, and only fifty-five others spent a year or more with him.[18]

The residency is now the expectation of all, a prerequisite to the coveted specialty status. During World War II, physicians with specialty training got better jobs and better pay in the armed forces. After the war, the demand for specialty training naturally increased. Established teaching hospitals could not accommodate all who applied. Non-teaching hospitals were quick to offer positions and were able to get accreditation for such training. In doing so, they acquired service personnel and status in their communities. Soon there were too many positions, and graduates of foreign medical schools came to fill them. As an illustration of the growth of residency training, in 1940 there were 5,097 graduates of American medical schools, 8,182 internship positions, but only 4,482 total residency positions. By 1950, there were 5,553 medical school graduates, 9,398 internship positions, and 18,669 total residency positions.[19] In the past ten or fifteen years there has been an effort to re-establish university control over such graduate training programs. The American Medical Association, the American Board of Medical Specialties, and the Association of American Medical Colleges cooperate in reviewing graduate training programs and in setting standards of competence in various subspecialty areas.[20] However, with the disappearance of the ward patient, the discontinuance of selective pyramiding to restrict the numbers of senior residents, and the development of a more senior elite of learners, the specialty fellow, the resident too has less responsibility in the course of training.

The social development of the young clinician has also changed markedly. Once single, unpaid, and almost entirely dependent on the economy of the hospital "household" and on older physicians for social contacts, house officers now lead a very different life: they are often married, they all receive salaries, and they generally spend a significant portion of their lives outside the hospital social system. Preparation for the medical profession is no longer a monastic novitiate, and the profession itself is no longer a brotherhood. This is true of other professions, but perhaps the change is more striking in medicine. There has also been a change in style and manner, perhaps in part the consequence of changing times, but arising also from the self-imposed isolation of the academic from society and the adoption of "academic manners." More casual dress, eating outside dining areas (often while in motion and aptly named grazing), inconsiderate manners, indulging in familiarity most apparent in the use of first names among strangers, all reflect changes in society at large but are more conspicuous in areas where social changes have been the most far-reaching, have become the most egalitarian, and have seen the greatest expansion in the numbers of people involved.

PROBLEMS RELATED TO CLINICAL EDUCATION

So what has all of this to do with Abraham Flexner? A great deal and, at the same time, not very much. There were forces at work in 1910 that would change society and, with it, medical practice and medical education. Who can have read the description of Edward VII's funeral in the opening chapter of *The Guns of August* without sensing at once the magnificence but also an imminent doom and the certainty of change? Who can be surprised that a society that produced almost contemporaneously *Mont-St.-Michel and Chartres* and *The Jungle* is diverse and in turmoil?[21]

Flexner was one of the players. His role was prominent, not crucial. He made a spectacular entrance with his report on *Medical Education in the United States and Canada*, the famous Carnegie Bulletin Number 4. Three years later, with the Rockefeller General Education Board paying the bill, he was accoucheur at the birth of the clinical full-time plan. His most significant accomplishments were in helping to take away control of hospitals and of medical education, especially clinical education, from the practicing medical profession and to bring it under the authority of academic bureaucracy, and in raising, at least in science subjects, the intellectual and academic requirements for medical school matriculation. Surely these things were going to happen as a consequence of multiple factors already in motion, but Flexner was able to crystallize them, to make them coalesce, to focus them into a recognizable movement with direction and momentum, and to shape the form of clinical education for the years that followed. He helped institutionalize the profession of medical educator. With that step have come both problems and benefits. It is not likely that another Abraham Flexner will appear to set today's problems right. Mr. Flexner's big stick, the money supply, is no longer in private hands. It is controlled now by two groups: private third-party insurers and the academic-federal bureaucracy.

Furthermore, the academic establishment (that is, the medical schools with their associated faculty) is no longer a fragmented collection of independent proprietary enterprises vulnerable to individual attack. It is in reasonably good control of its money supply through its peer-review network and because of its political and public relations activities. It can hardly be expected to entertain reforms that might jeopardize its very survival or change a structure that currently satisfies its beneficiaries. As Oliver Wendell Holmes put it more than a hundred years ago, it is unreasonable to expect a medical school to commit suicide for the sake of reform.

But should he return, what problems might a Flexner see? He would find new problems that had evolved from trends he himself had helped to initiate. The emphasis on science prerequisites is so high that we are often matriculating narrowly-educated students. We are attempting to train too many physicians with too few patients who stay in the hospital too short a time and who are too often unavailable because they are too sick or elsewhere having tests or treatments. Neither students nor house officers have the personal relationship or the responsibility that they formerly did, and both are so important to professional growth. The hospital, which Mr. Flexner did so much to bring under university control and to make central to clinical education, threatens to engulf its owners economically and professionally. Too many of those we train are heading for the more lucrative subspecialties in which they can limit their practice to pre-selected patients with problems amenable to specific and economically rewarding procedures or treatments, avoiding those with less well-defined, often more complex and time-consuming problems, especially those with social and psychological components to their illnesses. Those who do address these problems are forced by economics or by frustration to over-utilize technology.

Predictions of what is to come will be considered by other writers. The past has shown what predictions can be based on. The world of medicine now has three parts: the practitioner, the investigator, and the administrator; while there is some crossover, and while many espouse a dual or even triple role, most are lucky to excel at one.[22] How are we to modify the system to keep it in balance? The most important change in clinical education was the introduction of the clinical clerkship; now, for a variety of reasons, it is in jeopardy. The most important change in the search for new knowledge was the establishment of a funding system for career support that is now at risk because it has expanded beyond society's willingness to support it and requires expenditure of an unreasonable amount of clerical time in seeking and justifying that support. The development of a professional administrative cadre was beneficial, but like all such bureaucracies it is expanding exponentially and will consume too high a proportion of the resources.

However, the most important factor of all is the quality of those who choose medicine as a career. It is relatively easy to juggle the curriculum and devise appealing programs that attract funding from those who want to innovate, but what happens to the student at medical school is less important than what happened before medical school. Medicine is, in recent years, attracting a smaller proportion of our most talented young people. From 1910 to 1975 medicine became an elite activity in our society, partly because of what Mr. Flexner did, but that is now changing.

We honor still an image of a physician gone; the broad generalist who performs at the bedside, who exhibits those qualities Osler exemplified that have become anachronistic. Patients today do not call their doctors a few days after a consultation to ask what he or she has concluded; they call to find out "what the tests showed." It is not reasoned judgment they seek but the identity of that one test or several that they and many physicians have come to believe will give the answer to their problem. While there are such tests for an increasing number of man's ills, the majority of problems with which physicians do, or should, deal do not, or will not soon, have such easy solutions. Though we appear to have the best prepared, best selected, best trained medical profession of all time, there is room for concern. Are we training our physicians for the world they will live in? Are we training them to give the kind of care we want?

4

Women in Medicine Since Flexner

Mary Roth Walsh

For many, the Flexner Report remains a major explanation for the decrease in the numbers of women doctors in the early decades of the twentieth century. For example, Kenneth Ludmerer's highly acclaimed history of American medical education includes this comment: "Of all the oppressed groups, women suffered the most ironic setback. In the wake of the "Flexner Report," all but one women's medical college closed."[1] Since a number of other scholars have also viewed the "Flexner Report" as a crucial point in the history of women physicians, it seems useful to ask why so many writers have accepted the Flexner myth.[2]

In reality, the evidence is quite clear: the "Flexner Report" did not itself cause the women's medical colleges to close nor did it cause a decline in the number of women physicians. Both changes were well under way before Flexner began his study. In 1909, for example, the year before the publication of the "Flexner Report," fourteen of the seventeen women's medical colleges had already closed and the total number of women medical students, including those attending coeducational schools, had dropped to 921 from a total of 1,419 fifteen years earlier.[3]

Perhaps this misconception exists because scholars are unable to find another explanation for what happened in the early twentieth century to turn back the tide for women physicians. As I have documented elsewhere, the late nineteenth century in America was a relative golden age for women physicians. Compared to some other countries, relatively large numbers of women gained access to medical schools in this period, making the United States a leader in advancing the cause of women doctors. As it turned out, in spite of these initial gains, institutional barriers remained remarkably resilient in the first half of the twentieth century and they became the central force in limiting the number of women who entered medicine. As a result, there were fewer women physicians in Boston in 1950 than there had been in 1890 and this pattern was repeated in cities across the country.[4]

Sexism is not a simple phenomenon, however, and researchers have found it extremely difficult to tease out the causes as well as the solutions to the problems affecting women in American medicine. Some scholars still ignore the problems of sexism and play down its importance, somehow assuming that because they do not acknowledge it, it is not an important issue. William Rothstein, for example, has only two brief references to women in his 1987 history of American medical schools and the practice of medicine. Rothstein claims that medical education for women developed slowly in the nineteenth century and that there was an absence of overt sex discrimination in the period from 1950 to 1970, an assertion which is inconsistent with what we have learned about the topic in recent years.[5]

Unlike the period of the early 1970s, a growing literature on sex discrimination law now exists. Social and behavioral scientists have also demonstrated the extent to which sex bias determines both our perceptions and our behavior. The complex connection between patterns of sex discrimination and the determination of social policy is highlighted in a recent paper by Faye Crosby entitled "Sex Discrimination: How Can We Correct It If We Can't See It? And How Can We See It If We're Not Prepared to Correct It?"[6]

EARLY BARRIERS TO WOMEN IN MEDICINE

The evidence I have been able to gather on sex discrimination in the medical profession, from a variety of sources and spanning more than 150 years of history, suggests that from the very beginning the unwillingness to correct patterns of sex discrimination prevented some of the gatekeepers in medicine from seeing it in the first place. Certainly this was not true of all physicians and the problem was not limited to medicine or to men in our society. On the other hand, medical men were in a position to open the gates to women and their obduracy became the first barrier. Originally many men could not even conceive of women as physicians. Walter Channing, a professor of obstetrics at Harvard Medical School writing in the 1820s, claimed that it would be impossible for women to submit to the rigors of medical training. He reasoned that some of man's delicate feelings and much of man's "refined sensibility must be subdued" in the practice of medicine but the female psyche could never stand up to such a demanding career; womanliness would be completely destroyed. As Channing and most male physicians saw it, the female personality was entirely distinct from the male and this rhetoric reflects what historians have referred to as the "cult of true womanhood."[7]

But the subject to which every medical opponent of women was irresistibly drawn was the subject of the female reproductive system. "It was," one physician exclaimed, "as if the Almighty, in creating the female sex, had taken the uterus and built up a woman around it." To Horatio Storer, a gynecologist on the faculty of the Harvard Medical School who saw himself in direct competition with women surgeons, women were what they were "in health, in character, in her charms, . . . mind and soul because of her womb alone." Who could trust the great questions of life or death to one whose equilibrium varied from "month to month and week to week . . . up and down"? Storer claimed that menstruation led to "periodical infirmity . . . mental influences . . . temporary insanity" and it was a force to be reckoned with. In his opinion, women were crippled because of their biology, certainly more in need of medical aid than able to furnish it. Still, despite this opposition, women made slow but steady progress as the nineteenth century progressed. Women also began to invade the specialties of surgery and obstetrics.[8]

One of the outstanding obstetrician-gynecologists of this early period was Dr. Marie Zakrzewska, who founded the New England Hospital for Women and Children in 1862. After observing the statues of famous men in Westminster Abbey while on a trip to Europe in 1881, she wrote:

Will there ever be a monument to the first woman physician? We need such landmarks of civilization because the now living, as well as those who will live long afterward, need encouragement. The person who is covered by a monument is of no consequence, but the fact that a woman can work and make an impression upon civilization needs to be known to be remembered.[9]

When I began my research on women physicians, I found that Zakrzewska's hoped-for monument had not materialized. Even worse, much of the early history on women physicians had been distorted. Instead of descriptions of the incredible barriers confronting women physicians, a "blaming the victim" approach was used and women were depicted as being unable to meet the increased professional requirements for training emphasized in the "Flexner Report." In fact, as I have argued in my book and elsewhere,[10] women physicians welcomed the professionalization process with its carefully delineated medical prerequisites spelling out in detail the requirements for being a doctor.

Harriot Hunt, the first woman physician to practice in the United States, illustrates this point very poignantly. Hunt and her sister Sarah completed their medical apprenticeship with a husband and wife medical team and then began their practice as "female physicians" in Boston in 1835. Sarah Hunt practiced only a few years. Harriot described in her autobiography the problems women physicians encountered when they were shut out of medical schools and deprived of access to formal training. The fact that Elizabeth Blackwell is usually credited with being

America's first woman doctor reflects a historical double standard. Blackwell's status results from having been the first woman to have received a medical degree (in 1848), a standard which, applied to her male colleagues, would have sharply reduced the number of male doctors in the country.[11]

In New England, for example, from 1790 to 1840 in one of the few counties where we have demographic data on physicians, most male practitioners obtained their training by apprenticeship. In Worcester County, Massachusetts 73 percent of the physicians had not graduated from college, but still, as men, they could set up medical practices. Women who might have been interested in medicine in this preprofessional period were subject to numerous unwritten laws and customs which limited their visibility and obviously their practice of medicine. Even the apprenticeship experience was not equally open to women applicants, depending as it did on informal arrangements, usually with a male physician. Besides Harriot Hunt, there is little evidence that other women were able to become physicians through the apprenticeship route, though this was the norm for male physicians.[12]

THE BENEFITS OF PROFESSIONALIZATION

At this point, it is important to ask the question: did professionalization offer women their first real opportunity in medicine? The answer to this seems to be yes. If a medical degree was necessary, interested women could apply to medical colleges and if rebuffed, they could then establish their own. If medical society membership or a license was necessary, women could rise to meet the requirements and, if rejected, could raise the cry of injustice to gain support. In other words, it was easier to overcome known obstacles than to tilt at shadowy specters.[13]

One such known obstacle was the medical licensing exam. Women physicians regularly boasted how well they did on these tests. Official examination results categorized by sex do not exist, but women physicians, particularly those who attended women's medical colleges, were vigilant in this matter and occasionally compiled their own statistics. One study, published in the *Transactions of the Women's Medical College of Pennsylvania*, shows that only 4.9 percent of the graduates of the allopathic Pennsylvania and Baltimore schools and New York (homeopathic) school, which were the three remaining women's medical colleges, failed between 1901 and 1903. During the same period, 16.3 percent of the total graduates of the other medical colleges in the country failed the examinations.[14]

Women also made great strides in gaining access to established male medical schools in the closing decades of the nineteenth century. By the early 1890s, some forty medical colleges across the country, almost half of which were regular medical schools, had female enrollments of 10 percent or more. In a few cases, women accounted for more than half of the graduating classes.[15] The long struggle to gain access to the leading medical schools seemed assured when an enterprising group of women in Baltimore organized a campaign to endow Johns Hopkins University's long-delayed medical school on the condition that women be admitted on the same terms as men. Funds were raised in several cities and with the offer of a $500,000 endowment the financially beleaguered Johns Hopkins surrendered to the women's terms.[16]

THE EFFECTS OF THE DISAPPEARANCE OF WOMEN'S MEDICAL COLLEGES

Successes such as this contributed to the disappearance of the women's medical colleges because they encouraged the belief that separate islands of feminism were no longer needed. As Emily Blackwell noted when the New York Infirmary Medical School was absorbed by Cornell University Medical School in 1899: "It has now fulfilled its purpose and medical education may hereafter be obtained by women in New York in the same classes, under the same faculty, with the same clinical opportunities as men."[17]

In some ways, events at the Cornell Medical School were a microcosm of what was happening to women physicians in the years surrounding the publication of the "Flexner Report." Seventy women from the New York Infirmary entered Cornell in 1900 after it had absorbed the women's college. By 1903, the number of women students at Cornell had been reduced to ten. One way Cornell managed to cut the numbers of women was to create new obstacles for them. For example, the women students, unlike the men, were required to take their first two years of medical education at the Ithaca campus in upstate New York, some 250 miles from New York City. In response to a 1917 survey of medical education, the dean of Cornell's medical school admitted that the policy was deliberately adopted at the time to reduce the number of women medical students.[18]

Equally important, the absorption of the New York Infirmary cut short the teaching careers of a number of able young women faculty. Twelve years after the disappearance of the women's medical school, Cornell had yet to appoint a single woman to its major teaching staff.[19]

We know relatively little about the teaching faculty, either men or women, of most medical schools except in those few cases in which biographies have been written. Recent accounts of medical education, for example, provide only the sketchiest details about faculty character-istics.[20] The reasons that research on women faculty has been neglected are complex. Sexism and prejudice often made women invisible, and their teaching appointments were apt to be informal. Even a prominent woman such as Florence Sabin, a well-known professor at Johns Hopkins School of Medicine in 1911, was not eligible to vote on policy at the medical school.[21] When women were employed in off-track appointments, in "acting" positions, and as associates or lecturers, instead of in regular faculty slots, they were even less likely to appear in catalogues and medical school brochures because schools might not want to establish a formal precedent by making this information public.

Most nineteenth-century medical women and their friends viewed separate women's schools as a temporary expedient while they worked toward the long-term goal of gaining access to the coeducational medical schools. Nevertheless, the disappearance of women's medical schools has to be considered in any discussion of why the numbers of women doctors declined in the early decades of this century. To take just one case, the Women's Medical College of Pennsylvania graduated between 120 and 200 women each year between 1920 and 1968. These figures account for between one-fifth and one-third of all women graduates in that period.

Moreover a separate women's medical college was not just a matter of the number of graduates. The psychological significance of these schools was underscored by Dr. Alice Weld Tallant in an address in 1912 at the Women's Medical College of Pennsylvania, the longest surviving female medical school:

"Until I took my internship," she recalled, "I had never seen a woman operate, and I do not think those of you who have had your training in this (woman's medical) school can realize what it means to have never seen a woman doing that which to you seems second nature from your student days. It must be a great incentive to the student," she continued, "to see what women can do; it is almost inevitable, if you have never seen a woman doing anything, to think she cannot do it quite as well as a man, no matter how strongly you feel in favor of women."[22]

TWENTIETH-CENTURY OBSTACLES

Although it is hard to measure, the major problem in this historical period is that relatively few people, except for women physicians themselves, really valued the professional advancement of women in medicine. The first barriers that many medical women faced were within their own families. For example, the mother of Dr. Elizabeth Mosher, who attended the University of Michigan in the 1870s, claimed that when her daughter first broached the subject of going to medical school she said she would sooner see her shut up in a lunatic asylum. Dr. Dorothy Reed Mendenhall, who entered Johns Hopkins in 1900, later recalled that in all the years she was pursuing her degree in Baltimore, her aunt told her friends that Dorothy had gone South for the winter.[23]

Within the medical establishment, many opposed the advancement of women, some tolerated it, but few members of the medical establishment advocated the cause with enthusiasm. Most male physicians simply reflected the prejudices of the larger society. Consequently, the examples of the few men who did support women physicians and worked on their behalf stand out in the historical record. During the late nineteenth century, for example, women physicians were especially fortunate in attracting to their cause three of the most prominent physicians in Boston: Henry I. Bowditch, Samuel Cabot, and James Chadwick.

As Martin Duberman has noted, we know far too little about why people do anything, let alone why they do something as specific as joining a reform movement.[24] These three men differed in their areas of medical specialization and they ranged in age from Bowditch, who was seventy-one to Chadwick who was thirty-five years younger. The one thing all three men seem to have shared was a combination of personal and public success which enabled them to bear the tension connected with supporting a highly unpopular cause. Each man appears to fit Gordon Allport's definition of the mature personality: the ability to get outside one's self-preoccupation and involve oneself in abstract ideals. For Bowditch, who championed the first female applicant to the Massachusetts Medical Society, the women's struggle was an extension of the principles of the abolitionist movement he had joined in its infancy. Samuel Cabot had longstanding friendships with a number of women doctors and actively supported the New England Hospital for Women and Children. James Chadwick took the women's cause as his own and he not only carefully kept a scrapbook of clippings and letters to document their progress but he actively worked to gain allies for them.[25]

It is clear that medical leaders, with a few exceptions such as these, failed to supply what one would hope from them on this issue, that is, leadership. Though one can argue that they were merely men of their times, they clearly lacked the ability to appreciate the difficulties women faced. Even the medical reformers were blind to the problems of women in medicine. For example, Abraham Flexner, in 1910, casually dismissed the difficulties of women by noting that their choices in medical education were "free and varied." Flexner's visits to 155 medical schools in the United States and Canada, completed in a little more than a year, would challenge even a modern-day traveler who had access to planes and automobiles. In the first decade of this century, with poor roads and difficult travel conditions, Flexner must have made very fleeting site visits at individual schools. Considering the difficulties in recent decades of investigating sex discrimination and its impact on women's opportunities in professional education, it is understandable that he could not assess this phenomenon in the schools he visited. The information he gathered on women's medical opportunities was most likely based on anecdotes and comments from male physicians who were not particularly well informed about the realities women were experiencing. The aggregate statistics we have on medical school enrollments indicate that women were not as freely admitted to schools as Flexner argued. We also have considerable archival information on the obstacles women encountered once they did matriculate as students.[26]

When Flexner published his report in 1910, for example, more than half of the medical schools in the country did not accept women students.[27] Although some schools did open their doors to women for the first time in the years immediately following the "Flexner Report," those decisions did not arise from a real commitment to the equal education of women. Rather, they often reflected some combination of local events that tipped the balance. For example, Yale's decision to admit women for the first time in 1916 seems to have been stimulated by Henry Farnam, a Yale economics professor whose daughter wanted to enter medical school. When Farnam found out that the major obstacle to the admission of women was the $1,000 necessary to construct a separate women's bathroom, he offered to pay the bill himself. Yale accepted, the bathroom was built; and Louise Farnam went to medical school. It was a room that women students in the 1920s referred to as "the Louise Farnam memorial." The Farnam family got off cheaply. As previously noted, it cost women $500,000 in the 1890s to convince Johns Hopkins to open its doors to women.[28]

I should also point out that those schools that did open their doors to women did not open them very wide. Northwestern University Medical School admitted women in 1926 because Mrs. Montgomery Ward casually inquired, after her gift to Northwestern's endowment fund, whether the school admitted women. Unwilling to take any chances on Mrs. Ward's possible feminist sympathies, the university quickly decided to admit women and was rewarded handsomely when she doubled her original gift. But the school limited the number of women to four in each class. The university justified the number, which remained in effect with few exceptions until the 1960s, with the explanation that four was the number necessary for a complete dissecting team.[29]

Those interested in the medical education of women faced a new challenge in the twentieth century: the growing emphasis on postdoctoral medical training. But it was not these rising standards per se that threatened women. The problem lay in the fact that there were so few internships open to women. According to the 1921 *AMA Directory*, only forty of the 482 general hospitals approved for internships in the country admitted women interns. In other words, 92 percent of the available hospitals did not train women, however excellent a woman's medical school record. As late as the mid–1930s, twelve states had no hospitals available for women interns. In twelve other states, women medical school graduates could go to only one hospital for training.[30]

All of this meant that women had to limit their internship applications to a handful of hospitals. In 1925, for example, 50 percent of all women interns trained in nine widely separated hospitals, most of which were owned and operated by other women. One of these was located 5,000 miles away, in the Philippines![31] The result of this limitation was that women confronted a "systems effect." Women's inability to gain internships could be (and often was) used as a reason for not admitting them to medical schools. Opponents of the women argued: what profit was there in educating women doctors if they could not complete their critical post-graduate training?

The existence of quota systems in many medical schools also had a chilling effect on women's applications. Before the 1970s, most medical school officials publicly denied the existence of discrimination; but when guaranteed anonymity, they occasionally confirmed that female quotas existed. In 1946, the dean of one large eastern medical school acknowledged limiting the enrollment of women to six percent. As recently as 1961, another dean boasted that "Hell, yes, we have a quota," and "it's a small one. We do keep women out when we can. We don't want them here—and they don't want them elsewhere, either, whether or not they'll admit it." Another medical school spokesman remarked proudly, "Yes, indeed, we take women, and we do not want the one woman we take to be lonesome, so we take two per class."[32]

In fact, published information put out by the medical schools themselves is quite explicit about the existence of overt sex discrimination. For example, from 1959 to 1971 the AAMC handbooks on medical school admissions requirements included a separate information section for each school entitled: "Medical School Preferences," which was designed to guide the prospective student. Each school's policy regarding its preferences for applicants in terms of the sex, race, residence and age of applicants was described. Of the 88 coeducational medical schools listed in 1959, 28 percent stated in print that they preferred male students. In 1959, excluding the Howard and Meharry medical schools, only 10.5 percent of the schools admitted a racial preference. By 1963, 15 percent still expressed some bias against women applicants; 4.5 percent admitted a racial preference.[33] This does not mean that those schools that did not express sexual and racial preferences did not have them. It does demonstrate, however, that a significant number of medical schools during this period saw nothing wrong with expressing a preference for male candidates.

RECENT REFORMS

All this began to change in the 1970s with the rise of the feminist movement and the pressure of affirmative action. As a result, medical schools began to revise their discriminatory admissions policies, and the number of applications by women increased. Expectations of being accepted help to determine how many applicants apply to a particular school. Earlier, medical schools had helped to discourage potential female applicants through their admissions policies and subtle clues in recruitment and application procedures. When women perceived an improvement in their chances of being accepted, they increased their applications. This, in combination with federal guidelines requiring equal treatment, led to the dramatic increases of women students in the 1970s.

As a result, the blatant discrimination in recruitment and admissions procedures changed dramatically in the next few years. Schools began to openly welcome women. A University of Hawaii Medical School poster, for example, portrayed native Hawaiian, Asian, black and white women under the caption: "We're Going to be Doctors." The poster stated that "medicine is not for men only" and that the school "actively encourages women to apply."[34]

Other examples include a special recruitment publication entitled "Women in Medicine," published by Stanford University Medical School depicting a pregnant woman medical student ministering to a patient. The brochure contained this paragraph: "We're not being excluded now, and we're not dropping out. But far fewer women than men have been encouraged to apply to medical schools, including Stanford. And this is what we hope to change. We can soon expect about 25 percent female M.D.s but we need and want more."[35]

Aside from admissions changes, a great deal of the effort to combat sexism in medical education has been conducted on an ad hoc basis. Harvard Medical School, for example, published a student task force report in 1974 which identified a long string of discriminatory practices at the school such as role stereotyping, sexual innuendo, and ignoring female presence in a group situation.[36]

Attacks were also launched against medical textbook authors who used pictures of *Playboy* bunnies and other female models to enliven their presentations of scientific information. For example, Dr. Estelle Ramey led a successful battle to force the firm of Williams and Wilkins to withdraw their textbook, *The Anatomical Basis of Medical Practice*, from the market in 1972 because it contained pictures of nude females in seductive poses with captions such as:

We are sorry that we cannot make available the addresses of the young ladies who grace our pages. Our wives burned our little address books at our last barbecue get-together. If you think that once you have seen the backside of one female, you have seen them all, then you haven't sat in a sidewalk cafe in Italy where girl-watching is a cultivated art. Your authors, whose zeal in this regard never flags, refer you to [the following illustrations] as proof that female backs can keep an interest in anatomy alive.[37]

PROBLEMS STILL REMAINING

It is now about twenty years since the number of women admitted to medical schools began to rise rapidly. The sharpest increase took place in the 1970s. What has changed and what problems persist for the current crop of women medical students and physicians? The climate for women physicians has improved significantly in the past decade, but women will remain a minority within the profession for a long time to come. If the percentage of women medical students levels off at about 40 percent, not until the second decade of the twenty-first century will women constitute 25 percent of practicing physicians. Still, women physicians are no longer the anomalies they once were.

This is not to say that reservations about women in medicine have disappeared. In reviewing the recent literature I was surprised to see traces, albeit expressed in a more sophisticated and subtle way, of some of the issues that had "dogged the footsteps" of earlier medical women. One that I thought had been buried was the question whether women were constitutionally capable of pursuing a medical career. Admittedly, I found no echo of Dr. Horatio Storer's characterization in 1866 of menstruation as "temporary insanity."[38] Nevertheless, I did find a surprising number of articles which raised questions about the mental and physical capabilities of women physicians. This is not the place to do an exegesis of the literature, but I would like to cite just a few examples of the phenomenon. In an article entitled, "Suicide Among U.S. Women Physicians," the authors analyzed factors causing a higher suicide rate among the women. They calculated that "about 65 percent of American women physicians have primary affective disorders." Dismissing "role strain" as a possible cause of suicide, they concluded that there was a connection between affective disorders and the decision of women to pursue a medical career.[39]

Although I do not have space to carefully analyze this article, I refer interested readers to the letters to the editor in the December, 1979 issue of the *American Journal of Psychiatry*.[40] I would like to point out, however, that the original data reveal almost no gender differences in the suicide rates, which were 40.7 per 100,000 for female physicians and 38.1 for male physicians.[41] Perhaps, like beauty, some gender differences are in the eye of the beholder.

Another of the old arguments against women surgeons was that they lacked the strength to do the job. The more sophisticated modern version of this point of view can be found in a recent issue of the journal *Surgery*. After noting that right-handed residents scored higher on a number of tests, the authors traced the superior performance of male surgery residents at Loyola University to spatial and motor proficiency localized in the right hemisphere of the brain.[42] I was happy to read that the paper elicited the following response from a surgeon who supervised several of the residents from Loyola: "the best one we have seen yet is a woman who is right-handed [and] we have one left-handed woman for whom I predict stardom in academic surgery."[43] I'm not sure if this qualifies as a more "even-handed" evaluation of women's surgical skills. What is encouraging is that articles like this have resulted in responses from both males and females. Either women are no longer alone in their criticisms of these kinds of studies or editors feel compelled to publish more diverse letters of response.

There are, however, any number of unresolved problems related to the increasing number of women entering medical schools and the practice of medicine. If I had to choose one issue which constitutes a major dilemma for the woman physician and at the same time symbolizes medicine's difficulty in coping with women-related issues, it would be the problems surrounding pregnancy and parenting. In 1894, Dr. Gertrude Baille wrote in the *Women's Medical Journal* that many women physicians did not marry because they know "No woman can serve two masters." She argued that when a professional woman had a family, there was inevitable conflict between the two roles, and "Either her work or her family will feel the neglect."[44]

Today, women physicians do marry. Moreover, about two thirds of practicing women physicians have children. Almost one half of these have their first child during their training period, a time which usually coincides with the best physiological age for women to bear children, their late 20s and early 30s. Nevertheless, a study in the mid–1980s found that four-fifths of the residency programs surveyed had no policy on medical leave and most continue to treat pregnancy as a crisis rather than a predictable life event.[45]

Worse, some administrators seem to equate pregnancy during the training years with treason. For example, a recent article in the *Chronicle of Higher Education* reported that the chair of a gynecology department at a major medical school wrote a memorandum describing a resident's pregnancy as a "disservice" to herself and to her colleagues. His memo declared that her decision to have a baby before completing the three-year residency program raised the issue of women as "unreliable colleagues" and further challenged the idea of admitting women to residency programs in the first place. Indicating that we have made some progress, the dean of the medical school accepted the chair's resignation and likened his comments to those of "Attila the Hun."[46]

A more typical problem arising out of the failure to plan for residents' pregnancies is the concern of other residents who may have to take on extra work to cover the leave time that might be required during a pregnancy. Aware of this, many pregnant residents feel pressure to work as long as possible despite dangers to their own health and the fetus. Many hospital program directors still seem dedicated to treating internships and residency training as endurance tests. A case in point is a recent episode at Harvard. Dr. Maureen Sayres, director of the Harvard Medical School Office for Parenting, received a call from one of the residency program directors about a resident he described as suffering from post-partum depression. When Sayres investigated the case, she found that this woman resident had had to increase her weekly work schedule from the usual 100 hours to 118 hours to compensate for the fact that another resident had abruptly dropped out of the program.

The woman resident complied with the new schedule but found that she was constantly fatigued and saw nothing of her newborn son. After two months, she approached her training director for a reduction in hours and was told she was expected to carry her weight. Dr. Sayres' examination of the woman indicated that there was no postpartum depression, just "a normal physical and psychological response" to a work overload. What struck Sayres was that the structure of the residency training program transformed a normal response of exhaustion into a "pathological and psychiatric condition."[47]

The fact that Harvard Medical School has established an official Office for Parenting indicates that some programs are beginning to recognize the problems associated with pregnancy and child rearing. Efforts to take pregnancy into consideration have their own problems however. The issue of protective labor legislation for women has divided feminists since the passage of the nineteenth amendment. Even legal scholars are in deep disagreement on this issue. In the book *Gender Justice*, three legal policy experts dismiss maternity benefits as "the latest version of paternalism."[48] Nevertheless, I think that on balance, training programs which deal with pregnancy as part of a general set of policies related to parenting would meet a real need. It is interesting to note that there are five times more applicants for each place in the day care center in the Harvard Medical complex than for each place in the medical school.

The issue of parenting which is one example of how the special problems of women raise questions, for example about work hours and leave policies, that have relevance for all medical trainees. If the increased numbers of women in medicine do nothing more than force medical schools and hospitals to rethink the structure of their training programs, women will have made a major contribution to medicine.

5

Abraham Flexner and the Black Medical Schools

Todd L. Savitt

In 1900 a black student wishing to pursue a career in medicine could choose from ten schools in a variety of locations and settings (See Table 5.1). By 1920 this same student had only three choices and little assurance that any one of these schools would survive until graduation day. What had happened? The "Flexner Report," containing devastating comments on all but two of the black schools and negative statements about black physicians in general, appeared in 1910 and directly affected the fate of these schools. By 1923, only the two institutions he said deserved to exist, Meharry Medical College and Howard University Medical Department, remained. Those two schools, too, almost closed their doors as organized medicine and medical philanthropies pushed the educational reforms promoted by Flexner beyond the capacities of the black institutions to change. Between 1905 and 1920, black medical education passed through two crisis period: 1905 to 1912 and 1917 to 1918. Flexner was involved in both.

THE CONDITION OF BLACK MEDICAL SCHOOLS IN THE EARLY TWENTIETH CENTURY

Contemporaries classified black medical schools according to their origins as either missionary or proprietary (Table 5.1). Though some institutions in the North accepted a few blacks as medical students, no state, North or South, operated a medical school for blacks. In addition to establishing many colleges to educate freedmen after the Civil War, northern religious groups founded a small number of medical schools. For example, the Freedmen's Aid Society of the Methodist Episcopal Church oversaw the development of Meharry Medical College and Flint Medical School, and the American Baptist Home Mission Society allowed Shaw University to operate Leonard Medical School. Howard University and its Medical Department had Congressional backing but also received financial support from individual, non-sectarian donors. The proprietary schools, founded in every case by black physicians, had little if any outside funding.[1]

The precarious nature of their financial arrangements, whether overseen by white missionary groups or by enterprising black physicians, put all the black medical schools in a vulnerable position from the start. Most of the schools collapsed with the increased pressure for reform in the first decades of the twentieth century. Meharry, Howard, Leonard, Flint, Knoxville, and Louisville National were still struggling to survive and improve when American medicine "discovered" bacteriology, laboratories, public health, and the German education system. With the revitalization of the American Medical Association (AMA) and the Association of American Medical Colleges (AAMC) at the turn of the century and these organizations' relentless and application of pressure to improve medical education based on the new ideas in science and education, black medical schools found themselves caught in a paradoxical situation.[2] On the one hand, they saw the demand for their product—the M.D. degree—growing to the point where some of them could not accommodate all applicants. In 1907, President Charles F. Meserve of Leonard Medical School told Wallace Buttrick of the General Education Board (GEB), a Rockefeller family philanthropy, that his school had more applicants than places in each class, and more requests from towns for black physicians than graduates each year.[3] On the other hand, every black medical school faced mounting financial pressures as the demand for better trained professors, longer sessions, well-equipped laboratories, and clinical facilities drained limited resources. The proprietary schools had no sources of income other than student fees and perhaps a small investor or two. Theoretically, the missionary schools could raise funds from other parts of their universities, their home mission societies, or religious sect donors in the North.

In actuality, black colleges raised little excess funding to shunt into medical education and northern mission societies and individual donors at this time shifted priorities to such newer, more immediate problems as helping the large numbers of eastern and southern European immigrants who were moving into their cities. Moreover, black students generally came from poor families that could barely pay even the low tuition, fees, and living expenses of medical college, so the schools could expect little extra cash from that source. Few black physicians had succeeded well enough by the early twentieth century to support their alma maters, nor were black philanthropists able to do so.[4] State universities offered little for black citizens desiring a medical education. So the rising demand for black physicians and limited fund-raising opportunities caused problems for black medical schools at a time when they wished to encourage growth and modernization.

Table 5.1
Black Medical Colleges, 1865–1920

NAME	CITY	YEAR ORGANIZED	YEAR DISCONTINUED	AFFILIATION
Howard University	Washington, D.C.	1869		
Straight University Medical Department	New Orleans	1873 (?)	1874 (?)	American Missionary Assoc.
Lincoln University	Oxford, PA.	1870	1874	Presbyterian
Meharry Medical College	Nashville	1876		Methodist Episcopal
Leonard Medical School of Shaw University	Raleigh	1882	1918	Baptist
Louisville National Medical College	Louisville	1888	1912	Proprietary
Flint Medical College of New Orleans University	New Orleans	1889	1911	Methodist Episcopal
Hannibal Medical College	Memphis	1889	1896	Proprietary
Knoxville College Medical Department	Knoxville	1895	1900	Presbyterian
Chatanooga National Medical College	Chatanooga	1899	1908	Proprietary
State University Medical Department	Louisville	1899	1903 Merged with LNMC	Colored Baptist (Kentucky)
Knoxville Medical College	Knoxville	1900	1910	Proprietary
University of West Tennessee College of Medicine and Surgery	Jackson Memphis	1900 1907	1907 1925	Proprietary
Medico-Chirurgical and Theologiacl College of Christ's Institution	Baltimore	1900	1908 (?)	Proprietary

PRESSURES FOR CHANGE BEFORE FLEXNER

As historians have shown, Abraham Flexner did not inaugurate American medical education reform with his 1910 report.[5] He actually stepped into the middle of an era, put his imprint on it, and through his work with the GEB after 1912, influenced the way reforms were implemented. When Flexner began work for the Carnegie Foundation for the Advancement of Teaching in 1908, the Council on Medical Education (CME) had already evaluated all medical schools three times, twice using state medical licensing board results and once through personal visits. Dr. Arthur Dean Bevan (chair) and Dr. N. P. Colwell (secretary) had published in the *Journal of the American Medical Association* (*JAMA*) the failure rates of individual schools on board examinations and even a listing of acceptable colleges based on their classification scheme.[6] Though they did not publicize the reports stemming from their site visits, they sent these reports to the schools and to the state medical examining boards hoping to spur improvements at the poorer-rated institutions. The black schools fared badly in these three ratings. Their board failure rates in 1904 and 1905 all greatly exceeded 20 percent, the worst category,[7] and when the two years' scores were combined, each of the six schools with sufficient available data appeared in the bottom 30 percent of the 135 studied.[8]

After its establishment in 1904, well before Flexner's arrival, the CME promoted both higher entrance requirements and higher educational standards, making its appeals both to schools and to state regulatory boards.[9] Most black schools responded by lengthening their terms, improving hospital and laboratory facilities, and, at least in name, toughening entrance and graduation requirements.[10]

The CME had also noted, before Flexner, the cost to medical schools of needed changes and the necessity of obtaining outside funding for these reforms. A *JAMA* editorial in May 1907 announced that modern medical education now required two to three times the amount received in fees from each medical student. Proprietary schools, the editorial continued, simply did not possess the ability to raise and pay out such amounts; a large endowment from private sources or state support was needed to sustain a school. Medical education was changing for the better, it concluded, but too many schools lagged behind, unable to keep up with the rising standards.[11] At annual conferences on medical education, the CME began doing more than simply publicizing poor board scores and urging schools to improve; it proposed guidelines for an acceptable education program and wrote a model state medical practice act.[12]

So the CME's efforts before Flexner, though not directed specifically at black medical schools, in effect put them on notice. Administrators at these institutions understood the message and realized that the expense of change as well as the changes themselves threatened each school's existence. In June 1906 the CME sent a letter to every American medical school urging adoption of its proposal that all students take at least one year of college-level work in biology, chemistry, physics, and a foreign language before admission.[13] Acceptance of this plan would have immediately reduced the number of students at black medical schools because few young blacks went to college before starting their professional education. Furthermore, only a few black colleges offered such advanced courses and only a handful of white colleges admitted black students. Reduced enrollments in the black medical schools would have meant reduced income, a situation the black medical schools had to avoid, for both missionary and proprietary schools relied on student fees as the major source of funds. Not surprisingly, then, none of the black colleges responded positively to the AMA's request, though each year the number of white schools implementing the plan grew, as did the pressure for black schools to follow suit.[14]

The CME presented other reform ideas during these pre-Flexner years that threatened the black schools in particular. Arthur Dean Bevan, for instance, must have upset authorities at black schools with his comments about instructors, made at the April 1907 annual CME conference in Chicago. He alluded to some medical schools conducted by people respected in the profession, but imparting information and teaching the techniques of a former era. These institutions offered students little practical experience in the laboratory, the hospital ward, or the clinic, instead lecturing and quizzing them in the classroom.[15] Though catalogues of the black medical schools claimed to train modern physicians using modern techniques, other available information belies those statements. Leonard's faculty at this time, for instance, differed little from the faculty twenty-five years earlier, shortly after its opening. These local white practitioners, some highly respected in Raleigh and around the state, had trained early in the modern medical period. Some had not kept up with the new scientific ideas and educational innovations. With a tiny hospital open only during the school year and few laboratory facilities, Leonard could not really offer the best medical education to its students.[16] At Flint and Meharry, both supported in part by the Freedmen's Aid Society, many members of the predominantly black faculty were either recent medical graduates (usually of Meharry) with little practical experience, or graduates of many years ago who, because of race, often had not attended post-graduate courses. Faculty at the black proprietary schools consisted primarily of their own graduates, some just a year or two out of school.[17]

Chairman Bevan also attacked "medical schools conducted solely for profit" in his April 1907 address, calling them "a menace" and advocating their non-recognition.[18] Though the black proprietary schools had their failings, they seem not to have existed "solely for profit" and did turn out needed black practitioners. But the CME pressed hard to eliminate all proprietary schools and so put pressure on those run by and for blacks in this pre-Flexner period.

Finally, Bevan spoke quite critically of schools offering courses after four o'clock in the afternoon, when students with full-time jobs were no doubt tired from a day's work and had insufficient time to fit in full-length courses with laboratory and ward work. The AMA House of Delegates instructed the CME just two months after Bevan's address not to rate higher than Class C any medical college that offered evening courses.[19] Howard was then still offering night courses in Washington, D.C., where a strong demand for such a program existed.

So a year before Flexner even began his medical school survey, officials, faculty, and perhaps even students at black medical schools felt pressure to change their institutions' educational program. They could relate to their own colleges what Leonard President Meserve said of his: "A crisis has come in the life of the Leonard Medical School." The school, he felt, had no future if he could not find sufficient financial aid to upgrade it to meet the new educational demands.[20]

By December 1908 when Flexner began his study of medical education in the United States, three of the weakest (both financially and academically) black schools had closed their doors: the Medico-Chirurgical and Theological College of Christ's Institution in Baltimore, State University Medical Department in Louisville (merged with Louisville National Medical College), and Chattanooga National Medical College. Little is known about the first school; it apparently had no strong academic or financial basis and few graduates. The actual date of its closing is not clear, though it is not mentioned in AMA or AAMC records after 1908.[21] State University, despite its name, had no affiliation with the Commonwealth of Kentucky, but received its support from the state's black Baptist organizations. The university continued to train undergraduates and ministers after joining with Louisville National Medical College in 1903, eventually becoming Simmons College.[22] Almost nothing is known of Chattanooga National Medical College other than the fact that its founder named it after his alma mater, Louisville National Medical College. Presumably the Chattanooga school was a low-budget operation with little support from outside sources and too poor a reputation among prospective students and the state licensing board to survive even in so lax a state as Tennessee, where medical school charters and licenses to practice medicine were easily obtainable.[23] Three of the seven remaining black schools, the University of West Tennessee and Knoxville Medical College (both proprietary) and Leonard Medical School (Baptist) received rating of less than 50 percent from the CME in June 1908.[24] The

CME also recommended that state examining boards withdraw recognition from these institutions.[25]

FLEXNER'S EVALUATION OF BLACK MEDICAL EDUCATION

Black medical education, therefore, already faced hard times when Flexner completed and published his report in 1910.[26] The Report only worsened the situation by: (1) announcing the existence of black medical schools that turned out practicing black physicians; (2) describing the good and bad points of these schools and advocating improvements or closings just as with the white schools; (3) reflecting an outlook about black medical education that the AMA readily accepted and applied in its formulation of education policy; and (4) revealing negative white attitudes toward black physicians during an era of increasing racial tension.

Until the "Flexner Report," organized medicine said little directly to or about the black medical schools. Though the CME, almost from its establishment in 1904, issued annual reports, articles, and commentaries on medical education in *JAMA*, never in the decade-and-a-half of major medical education reform did *JAMA* ever openly discuss the issue of medical education for blacks. Women's medical education received a passing reference in each annual education issue and an occasional article. Black schools received no notice other than "colored" listed next to their names in tables, and one-sentence statements when one of them received a gift, completed a building, or closed. Even state medical journals of the period rarely acknowledged the presence of black schools within the state's borders.[27] The "Flexner Report," with its description of each of the seven existing black institutions and a less-than-two-page discussion of black medical education problems, at least documented the almost invisible presence of black medical schools.

But the "Flexner Report" also harmed the black cause by portraying as deficient black medical education in general and five of the seven black medical schools in particular. It said little good about the three proprietary schools—West Tennessee, Louisville National, and Knoxville—or two of the missionary schools affiliated with universities—Flint and Leonard. It did praise the "small and scrupulously clean hospital of 8 beds" at Louisville National.[28] But it also noted the "meager equipment for chemistry, pharmacy, and microscopy" and the "bare . . . rooms" at West Tennessee,[29] the absence of laboratory or clinical facilities at Knoxville[30] and the paucity of laboratory materials at Leonard[31] and Flint.[32] Flexner's criticisms were harsh ("The catalogue of this school [Knoxville] is a tissue of misrepresentations from cover to cover"),[33] frank

("Of the three negro schools in the state [Tennessee], two are without merit"),[34] chiding ("The school [Knoxville] occupies a floor above an undertaker's establishment"),[35] sarcastic ("It was stated by a student that twice between October 1 and January 28 'a few students were taken to the Knoxville College Hospital' "),[36] and biting ("Laboratory facilities [at Leonard] . . . comprise . . . a slight chemical laboratory, and a still slighter equipment for pathology").[37] Sometimes he allowed the mere statement of facts without comment to convey his message: "The school [Flint] controls a hospital of 20 beds, with an average of 17 patients monthly, and a dispensary with an average daily attendance of one or two";[38] "There is a dispensary [at West Tennessee], without records, in the school building."[39] Flexner's reports on these five schools told readers that black students, and, by implication, current black practitioners who had graduated from these schools, did not receive an adequate medical education. He even stated at one point: "Of the seven medical schools for negroes in the United States, five are at this moment in no position to make any contribution of value to the solution of the [negro health] problem above pointed out. They are wasting small sums annually and sending out undisciplined men, whose lack of real training is covered up by the imposing M.D. degree."[40]

The Report did more than describe poor conditions at black medical schools. It prescribed a limited role for black physicians in their practices and hinted that black physicians possessed less potential and ability than their white counterparts. The tone of Chapter XIV, "The Medical Education of the Negro,"[41] illustrated well how, in the world of medicine as in so many other aspects of American life at the time, whites attempted to discount, dominate, and disvalue blacks. Flexner's choice of pronouns in this chapter presumed that blacks would not read it. He began with a provocative statement: "The medical care of the negro race will never be wholly left to negro physicians." His second sentence explained this assertion, by claiming that whites had to teach the black physician "to feel a sharp responsibility for the physical integrity of his people." Black doctors, according to Flexner, lacked responsibility enough to take over full care of their own people, but white doctors possessed that sense. Furthermore, "The practice of the negro doctor will be limited to his own race." Flexner's reasoning for such comments became clearer as he next explained how educating black physicians would also serve white interests in preventing the spread of black diseases among whites. He was clearly writing for a white audience when he concluded, "The negro must be educated not only for his sake, but for ours." To protect the nation's overall health, the responsibility of "educating the [black] race to know and to practice fundamental hygienic principles" fell naturally to the black doctor. Thus, "a well-taught negro sanitarian will be immensely useful." So Flexner not only limited the role of black physicians to caring for other blacks, but further restricted it to matters of public health.

Where did black medical schools fit in Flexner's scheme? They had two missions: first, to offer "the more promising of the race ... a substantial education in which hygiene rather than surgery ... is strongly accentuated"; second, to

imbue these men with the missionary spirit so that they will look upon the diploma as a commission to serve their people humbly and devotedly, away from large cities [in] the village and [on] the plantation, upon which light has hardly as yet begun to break.

If Flexner spelled out in more detail how to implement a program to accomplish these goals for black medical education, so different in many ways from the more research- and practice-oriented program for whites described in the rest of his report, he must have done so orally. None of his extant letters to the black medical schools or his published writing discussed these matters.

The two medical schools that Flexner believed to be suited for training black physicians were Meharry and Howard. He admired Meharry founder George W. Hubbard's skill at marshalling slender resources and building his school into a credible institution with good laboratory facilities and a small but well-managed endowment. Meharry lacked only a larger hospital and dispensary. Howard, with its ties to the federal government through a small annual appropriation and the use of Freedmen's Hospital, had its future "assured." Both schools, Flexner knew, needed "developing," and both were "unequal to the need and the opportunity" as they then existed. He urged religious and philanthropic organizations as well as individuals to concentrate their efforts on these two institutions and not to waste separate small amounts of money on the other five schools.[42] Flexner's recommendation on medical education for blacks in 1910 was to close the five "ineffectual" schools and encourage their supporters to donate time and money toward building Howard's and Meharry's programs.

THE INFLUENCE OF THE "FLEXNER REPORT"

In the end, Flexner's black medical school plan prevailed. Only Howard and Meharry survived the reform era, though both continued to train a full range of medical practitioners rather than sanitarians for rural blacks. Of the five other institutions, three closed within two years of the Report, one fought on doggedly for another eight years, and one proprietary school defiantly remained open till 1923, though unrecognized by most state licensing boards. Knoxville Medical College, criticized severely by Flexner, closed the same year the Report was published. The following year, Flint Medical College, sponsored by the same Freedmen's Aid Society that supported Meharry, shut down after twenty years. Flint's president explained that the CME's increasingly intense campaign for improved standards, and the school's lack of money to make the necessary changes, forced its closing.[43] Louisville National Medical College lost its accreditation from the Kentucky State Board of Health and closed in 1912.[44] The influence of the "Flexner Report" can be seen in the demise of each of these schools.

Few if any blacks responded directly to the Report in writing, though physicians and educators must have discussed it. The Committee on Medical Education of the National Medical Association (NMA)—black counterpart to the AMA—had considered the problems of black medical schools in 1908 and 1909 after the publication of state board scores in *JAMA*, but remained silent (at least in writing) on the "Flexner Report" and medical education in general after 1910. This committee had no power to implement education policy at black medical schools; it simply advised NMA officers and members of medical education matters and made recommendations for improvements. The committee had recognized the weaknesses of the several black colleges even before Flexner and wished to avoid public embarrassment over them. That, unfortunately, was no longer possible.[45]

In 1912, the end of this first crisis period, only four black schools remained. One of these, West Tennessee, was isolated from the others until it closed in 1923, its president taking an independent course.[46] Howard and Meharry, the two schools of which Flexner spoke positively, seemed to have bright futures, leaving only Leonard to prove itself worthy and secure a firmer position.

The "Flexner Report" did not conclude an era of medical reform; it appeared in the midst of one. Medical education standards continued to change, to improve, pushed along by the schools themselves, the AMA, the AAMC, state licensing boards, and by two major funding agencies, the Carnegie Foundation for the Advancement of Teaching and the GEB. The remaining black schools still faced difficult times. Howard and Meharry had received A ratings from the AMA in the second round of visits (the Flexner visits of 1909 to 1910), though in a special category called "Medical Schools for the Colored Race."[47] They had to keep up with the latest innovations to retain their positions. Leonard, rated C, had to catch up.

The "Flexner Report" had brought attention to seven black medical schools: their presence, their needs, their shortcomings, and their potential. Three could not change sufficiently, and closed. The remaining schools had to prove themselves. But no one in the white medical establishment, not even Flexner, who wanted Howard and Meharry to endure, helped the schools through this next crisis period until one more had closed and the other two were about to follow suit.

THE SEARCH FOR FUNDING

On February 21, 1910, Howard University President Wilbur Thirkield acknowledged receipt of an advance copy of Flexner's assessment of his medical school: "We are deeply gratified by this favorable representation of the equipment and work of the school." He told Henry S. Pritchett, president of the Carnegie Foundation, that Howard would immediately require of all its freshmen applicants one year of college-level science.[48] Three months later Edward Balloch, medical dean, submitted his annual report to President Thirkield, telling him of the faculty's pleasure with the new admissions requirements but concern at the anticipated decline in enrollment and loss of revenue from student tuition. Because Howard relied on fees for most of its income, plus a small allowance from the federal government, Balloch knew that trouble lay ahead. Only by the extraordinary efforts of the school's secretary-treasurer, the underpayment of faculty salaries, and strict economy of educational expenditures, did the Medical Department break even each year. Student fees just covered costs. But, Balloch continued, it was not fair to pay the faculty so little or to provide them with so few supplies and so little equipment. The Medical Department needed at least $10,000 over tuition and fees the following year to pay for the cost of education. What Howard really needed was a half-million dollar endowment. Securing one "should be given precedence over everything else."[49]

Within months Thirkield wrote a letter to Andrew Carnegie, reminding him of his expression of interest in Howard University Medical Department at the recent Carnegie Library dedication on campus.[50] Undeterred by Carnegie's quick response that Howard was worthy, but that he had given them $50,000 for the library the previous year and the government already provided annual financial support,[51] Thirkield held further discussions with Carnegie's personal secretary. In May of 1911 he submitted an ambitious proposal for $200,000 to erect and equip a new building for the medical school. This time he enclosed references from Dr. William Henry Welch of Johns Hopkins, Pritchett of the Carnegie Foundation, President William Howard Taft, and Dr. Woodward of the Carnegie Institution, attesting to the value and importance of this investment. He included a fact sheet illustrating the school's need for buildings, salaries for full-time professors, and other budget items. Then, as President Meserve of Leonard Medical School had stated just a few years earlier in an appeal for funds, Thirkield explained that the Howard Medical Department "has reached a crisis in its affairs."

On the one hand, it is confronted with the necessity of providing medical education for colored students which shall comply with modern standards; on the
other hand is the absolute impossibility of providing such education when the
income is derived from fees alone.

Taking his cue from Flexner's Report, Thirkield informed Carnegie that
Howard "trains men of science, especially versed in the problems of
sanitation and preventive medicine." The work of its graduates will improve white health as well as black because many diseases are transmitted
from one race to the other.[52] Despite these appeals and others over the
next few years, no dollars from the Carnegie fortune found their way
to Howard Medical School.[53]

Dr. Hubbard of Nashville also appealed to Carnegie for $20,000 to
build a hospital. Flexner had urged its construction in 1910 to make
Meharry a first-rate medical school. Carnegie agreed, and donated
$10,000 on condition Hubbard raise the rest. This he did, and in 1913
the G. W. Hubbard Hospital was dedicated.[54] But Meharry's further
appeals, like Howard's, for larger sums or for an endowment, elicited
similarly negative responses. Andrew Carnegie finally told Pritchett, who
had urged funding, "If we start helping medical colleges for colored
people we cannot discontinue." Their needs, he felt, were too great, and
their allies who might help in the funding too few.[55]

The needs of black schools *were* great—too great for small philanthropists or religious outreach boards like the Freedmen's Aid Society
or the American Baptist Home Mission Society to manage. Yet the Carnegie Foundation, the philanthropy that had supported the investigation
that ultimately encouraged continuation of Meharry and Howard, refused financial assistance to these schools. In 1912 Flexner moved to the
other large, education-oriented philanthropic organization in the United
States, the GEB. Black medical school officials wrote to both Flexner and
Pritchett, hoping that the personnel change signaled a policy change as
well, but the GEB and Carnegie Foundation turned them down or delayed action for several years.[56]

A SECOND CRISIS PERIOD

Between 1912 and 1918 the situation worsened for the black schools.
Leonard could not get the ear of any funding agency after the GEB
gave it a tiny amount toward a new hospital in 1910.[57] In 1914 the school,
despite its high admission standards and reasonably good laboratory
facilities, of necessity dropped its clinical program in exchange for a B
ranking from the CME.[58] Earlier that same year Meharry lost its A rating
and received a reprimand from the CME representative who visited the

school. A number of problems had been identified: the faculty consisted of only three full-time and twenty-four part-time instructors for 354 medical students; the school's enforcement of student entrance standards could not be verified from existing records; medical, dental, and pharmacy students took classes together; the new hospital, with fifty-eight beds, had only twenty-three occupants at the time of the visit and averaged only thirty; the outpatient department served only six to eight patients per day; no medical library, medical museum, or modern teaching tools such as reflectoscopes or stereopticons were available for student instruction; laboratories were poorly equipped; no course was offered in pharmacology; the curriculum was only partially graded—first- and second-year students took classes together, as did third- and fourth-year. To that time, the inspector stated in his report, Meharry had retained a Class A rating because it was a black school. After each previous inspection, investigators had told school authorities of existing problems and how to correct them. Many of the deficiencies could have been corrected at little expense. Because Howard University upheld proper entrance requirements (it had just begun insisting on two years of college courses) and offered a strong education program, the CME need not keep Meharry "in a classification where it clearly does not belong." So the CME voted to reduce Meharry to a B ranking.[59] Medical education for blacks seemed to be deteriorating.

The CME, in addition to rating schools, campaigned to tighten state licensure requirements. More and more states began insisting on basic college science courses,[60] or even two years of college, as entrance standards for their medical schools or as prerequisites to taking licensure exams. Some states even refused licenses to graduates of class B and C schools.[61]

The black schools continued to appeal for help from Pritchett at Carnegie and Flexner at the GEB. Neither man ignored the problem, but both found their efforts thwarted or delayed by their own or other agencies. They tried to convince their respective boards to fund black medical education between 1912 and 1916, but neither foundation would be pushed too quickly.[62] Not until December of 1916 did the two agencies combine forces and offer Meharry, as a stopgap measure, $15,000 a year so that it could remain open, but still without an endowment.[63] As Flexner observed Howard's and Meharry's struggles to maintain their programs, he worried that they, and in fact all medical schools in the South, ought not be pushed into radical changes too quickly lest they be forced to close unnecessarily. They should not, he believed, be compared to white northern schools, but rather should be permitted to make improvements based on a less compressed timetable. Flexner strongly disapproved of the CME's constant pressure on Meharry to improve. In late 1914, he feared that Meharry would "be choked" if the CME forced too many changes too quickly on the black schools. But the CME persisted in spite of Flexner's protests.[64]

In fact, the schools *were* being choked. They were caught in a power squeeze between, on the one hand, two large foundations that put white medical educational needs above black, and on the other, a powerful medical organization that refused to recognize the special needs of black medical schools and black doctors. The crisis peaked in the fall of 1917. None of the three black medical schools was healthy, and Leonard was about to collapse. Hubbard presented the problems of black medical schools to the annual meeting of the Southern Medical Association, which passed a resolution urging the AMA to take action to save the schools.[65] Dr. Aaron McDuffie Moore, a Leonard graduate and dedicated Durham, North Carolina physician, headed a committee of the National Medical Association that drew up an eloquent and desperate "Appeal for Medical Education for Negroes" which he sent to the AMA, the GEB, and the Carnegie Foundation.[66] Meharry and Leonard officials asked the CME for reinspections and A ratings, lest they lose recognition with the licensure boards of several southern states. The CME responded that it would happily re-evaluate the schools, but that without endowments Leonard and Meharry could not improve their education programs in any meaningful and permanent way. Nor could the CME compromise its standards for some schools without jeopardizing its own credibility. The problem was really out of its hands. State licensing boards and medical colleges themselves were increasing the pressure to raise standards.[67] Dr. N. P. Colwell, secretary of the CME, did personally appeal to Flexner and Pritchett to give endowments to the black schools, asserting that the GEB and Carnegie Foundation were doing these colleges "a grave injustice" by withholding funds.[68] He had on February 4, 1918 already made these statements publicly in an address to the CME conference of 1918, which was later published.[69] Flexner and Pritchett responded hotly and frankly, asking Colwell to consider "how far this injustice is due to the action of the Council." They felt the black schools were making "good progress under the normal pressure of improvement" and did not need CME's harsh prodding.[70]

By May 1918 Dr. Moore and others were desperate. Leonard faced imminent closing, and black doctors attending recent state association conventions were "very much depressed" over the situation there and at Meharry. Using words that illustrate the stature Flexner had achieved in medical education circles, Moore wrote to him: "We are making our final appeal to you as the most potent representative of the medical profession in America and also as the Financial Agent whose word is final on such matters. We regard your Board [GEB] as an equalizing agency," since tax money in the South is spent on educating white physicians and none is spent on black medical education.[71] Flexner, however, deflected the arrow of blame back at the CME and Colwell. Accusations and denials again flew back and forth. Colwell labeled the situation a "so-called crisis," claiming that recent actions by Florida, North Carolina, and Virginia to deny recognition to Class B institutions had "suddenly awakened Meharry and Leonard to the importance of seeking a Class A rating—a rating which they have been content to do without for several years."[72] Interestingly, in the midst of these battles over the fate of black medical schools, fought between organized white medicine and organized white philanthropy, the principal leaders on both sides found one point on which they agreed: that "high-grade white schools such as Columbia and the University of Pennsylvania" needed funding on a large scale before the black schools.[73]

In the end, no agency acted to save Leonard, which closed before the 1918–1919 school year began.[74] The annual $15,000 joint Carnegie Foundation/GEB appropriation kept Meharry alive for another year until the two foundations could finally agree on a $300,000 grant, contingent on Meharry's raising $200,000 more.[75] Howard, the school with the most promise in 1910, staggered along without significant philanthropic funding until the early 1920s, as Pritchett and Flexner favored Meharry.[76] The first two decades of the twentieth century ended with three black medical schools still open: West Tennessee existing precariously as an unrecognized proprietary institution, Meharry and Howard with small endowments, and none with an assured future.

Abraham Flexner worked closely on the problems of medical education for blacks from 1908, when he began his study for the Carnegie Foundation for the Advancement of Teaching and the AMA, through the next decade. He believed only Howard and Meharry possessed the potential for success in the medical education system he envisioned, and argued for their survival at the expense of the other five. Those five did close, three, it appears, as a direct result of his 1910 report, one (Leonard) despite his attempts to ease the CME's pressure on it, and one (West Tennessee) for other reasons. His strong efforts to provide funding for Meharry helped save that school from closing. Flexner had a great impact on black medical education in the early twentieth century.

BLACK MEDICAL EDUCATION TO MID-CENTURY

From 1920 to 1950, the two remaining black medical schools continued their struggle for existence in the white medical world, one emerging stronger than the other. A black student entering either school during these years might still have wondered, as had students in 1900, whether the school would survive until graduation day. By the 1930s, though, Howard was in a less precarious position than Meharry. Organized medicine and large philanthropies continued to exert influence over the schools.

For Meharry in 1921, the first priority was obtaining an A rating from the CME. Flexner convinced a reluctant CME in 1922 to raise Meharry's ranking after it had twice in two years refused to do so. But Meharry was still not, in the opinion of many, an A school. As one recent historian characterized Meharry during this period: "laboratory facilities were grossly inadequate; instructors were overworked, poorly paid, and undertrained; library resources were virtually non-existent; and students were indiscriminately admitted."[77] Its president, John J. Mullowney, Hubbard's successor, mismanaged the institution and generated much ill-will among faculty, staff, and within Nashville's black community. The GEB, under Flexner's influence, poured millions of dollars into the school's budget (about $8,000,000 between 1916 and 1949), and became involved between 1933 and 1938 in the movement to remove Mullowney and appoint Edward Turner of Chicago. Turner did much to improve the school in a short time, saving Meharry's A rating in 1938. Money problems continued to plague the school through the 1940s. Announcements by the GEB and other philanthropies during that decade that they would soon cease making contributions to Meharry plunged the institution into another financial crisis at the dawn of the Civil Rights Era.[78]

Howard also faced financial problems between 1920 and 1950, but of a different sort. Because the United States Department of the Interior provided funds for Howard's operating budget and free teaching use of Freedmen's Hospital, adjacent to campus, large philanthropies like Carnegie and the GEB saw Howard's maintenance as a government responsibility. In 1920 Howard desperately needed help, not with clinical education (Freedmen's Hospital served that aspect well), but in the basic sciences. As Flexner characterized Howard's wants in a 1920 memorandum to the GEB, "The laboratory branches are starved for support and equipment."[79] He urged the GEB to contribute $250,000 toward a $500,000 endowment and to make funds immediately available for hiring basic science faculty and for laboratory equipment. This time GEB agreed and donated about $700,000 over the next twenty-one years. This amount, joined with increased government appropriations, a gift from the Julius Rosenwald Foundation, and donations from black and white citizens across the country, provided Howard, by the 1940s, with an improved physical plant and faculty and a small but solid endowment fund. Strong leadership during this period from President Mordecai Johnson, and from Numa P. G. Adams, first black dean of the medical school, placed Howard in a strong position to face the new problems of the Civil Rights Era.[80]

By 1950, Howard and Meharry together were graduating about one

hundred black physicians annually, and white medical schools were graduating a total of about ten to twenty more. Depression had taken its toll
on potential black physicians who could not afford to attend medical
school. The number of black practitioners in the United States dropped
five percent between 1932 and 1942, while the number of white physicians increased 12 percent. The need for more black physicians remained strong, but the capabilities of the two medical schools that trained
black students remained limited. The many applicants rejected from
Howard and Meharry in the late 1940s had few options at other medical
schools.[81] Flexner, in the early 1920s, had saved the two schools he
thought worth saving. But the demise of the other black medical schools
had created problems Americans were just beginning to face in the
1950s.

6

The Fate of Sectarian Medical Education

Norman Gevitz

Medical historians have found themselves in a quandary when it comes to placing osteopathic medicine within the context of medical education in the United States during the twentieth century. Either they make no mention at all of the subject, or they add the caveat that for the purpose of their study osteopathic medicine will not be discussed.[1] Indeed, unless one reads the "Flexner Report," one would never guess from the vast literature dealing with its significance or relative impact that Abraham Flexner surveyed all D.O.-granting institutions as well as M.D.-granting schools. I believe that a consideration of the development of osteopathic medical education is important for a full understanding of the evolution of American medical education in the first part of this century, as it provides a comparative example through which the general processes of educational change and the internal and external pressures for reform can better be appreciated. The major question that I will concern myself with is: why did M.D.-granting sectarian schools disappear and osteopathic colleges survive?

The first osteopathic school was established in Kirksville, Missouri in 1892, by the founder of the movement, Andrew Taylor Still (1828–1917). Still, a frontier doctor trained through the apprenticeship system common before the Civil War, had become dissatisfied with the therapeutics of his day. Influenced by the doctrines of magnetic healing and bonesetting, he came to believe that disease was primarily due to misplacements of the spinal vertebrae which affected the nerves regulating the flow of blood throughout the body. Thus, to eliminate disease, one needed to correct these spinal "lesions" through physical manipulation. Although the first class at his institution received instruction only in anatomy and osteopathic diagnosis and therapy, Still soon included the other basic sciences as well as minor surgery, obstetrics, and the use of a limited number of drugs (antiseptics, anesthetics, and antidotes). His goal was to produce well-rounded general practitioners. Soon other schools were founded and by the turn of the century the movement was reasonably well established.[2]

Osteopathy was following in the footsteps of the older medical sects of homeopathy and eclecticism. Homeopathy was founded by a German physician, Samuel Hahnemann (1755–1843), who believed that drugs that produce symptoms in healthy persons will cure those symptoms in a sick person by creating an artificial disease which substitutes for the real one. He also argued that the more diluted the dose the stronger the drug's actions.[3] Eclecticism was launched by Wooster Beach (1794–1868), who like Hahnemann rejected orthodox medicine's reliance upon bloodletting and other heroic depletive measures. Beach sought to substitute native American botanical remedies for mineral drugs.[4] Each of these sects had established M.D.-granting schools by the 1840s and each movement continued to maintain colleges into the twentieth century.

FLEXNER AND THE SECTARIAN SCHOOLS

The impetus behind the inclusion of osteopathic medical education in Flexner's study seems to have come from Henry Pritchett, head of the Carnegie Foundation. He and Flexner attended a meeting on December 28, 1908 with the members of the American Medical Association (AMA) Council on Medical Education (CME) to discuss the impending survey. According to the minutes,

President Pritchett related his experiences with an osteopath in a small Colorado town, making his lame leg an excuse for calling as a patient but seeking information about the osteopath's methods and what kinds of cases he treated. It was found he was treating even adenoids and appendicitis. Therefore, it was clear that osteopaths (at least this one) were diagnosing the same diseases which physicians were called upon to treat, therefore osteopaths should have the same training in fundamentals.[5]

While members of the CME asked Pritchett about his encounter, they expressed no interest in including osteopathic education in the Carnegie Foundation study. Thus, it was apparently at Pritchett's urging rather than the CME's that Flexner investigated the osteopathic colleges.

Flexner excoriated almost all the existing homeopathic, eclectic, and osteopathic schools for poor standards, and made no allowance for the survival of any of them in his reconstruction plans for medical education.[6] Nevertheless, he reserved some of his sharpest criticism for osteopathic institutions. Flexner observed, "Let it be stated with all possible emphasis that no one of the eight osteopathic schools is in a position to give training as osteopathy itself demands." The basic sciences, he noted, were poorly presented. The teaching of anatomy was in Flexner's words "fatally defective." Most of the students' time was spent listening to lectures—there being too few cadavers available for dissection. Flexner noted, "A small chemistry laboratory is occasionally seen. At Philadelphia it happens to be in a dark cellar. At Kirksville, a fair-sized room is devoted to physiology and bacteriology; the huge classes are divided into bands of thirty-two, each of which gets a six-weeks course following the directions of a rigid syllabus, under a teacher who is himself a student." At the Kansas City college there were practically no laboratories; at Des Moines, instead of laboratories there were only "laboratory signs"; and at Chicago, the process of rebuilding its laboratories went on "without in the least interfering with its usual pedagogic routine."[7]

Flexner believed clinical instruction was no better. He noted, "The osteopath cannot learn his technique and when it is applicable except through experience with ailing individuals. And these for the most part he begins to see only . . . after receiving his D.O. degree."[8] Indeed, bedside training was very limited or non-existent. Kirksville had the largest hospital, only fifty-four beds, while three schools—Des Moines, Kansas City, and Los Angeles—had no hospitals at the time of his visit. Outpatient contact was similarly restricted. Each of the colleges, he maintained, operated a pay clinic staffed by the faculty in which student participation seems to have been limited to charity cases.

In characterizing the entire educational program, Flexner declared, "The eight osteopathic schools now enroll some 1,300 students who pay some $200,000 annually in fees. The instruction furnished for this sum is inexpensive and worthless." He declared that no school had any full-time teachers, and the school owners were either pocketing most of the fees or using the funds for buildings.

No effort is anywhere made to utilize prosperity, as a means of defining an entrance standard or developing the 'science.' Granting all that its champions claim, osteopathy is still in its incipiency. If sincere its votaries would be engaged in critically building it up. They are doing nothing of the kind.[9]

As one might expect, the osteopathic community did not respond favorably to Flexner or his survey. Similar to administrators of some M.D.-granting colleges, deans of osteopathic schools claimed that Flexner spent as little as a single hour in their institutions. They attacked him for alleged factual errors and gross misinterpretations. The *Journal of Osteopathy*, based at the Kirksville school, took him to task for declaring there was not a full-time teacher in any osteopathic college. It noted, "In this Flexner either lied or didn't take the trouble to find out the truth, as the whole profession knows; in either case, he is unfit for the position he holds. Possibly we may not understand what Mr. Flexner means by a 'full-time teacher.' It is true that some of the teachers at Kirksville do not spend more than fourteen to sixteen hours a day in school work, but they offer as an excuse that they must eat and sleep a little." The journal concluded, Flexner "came to find fault. He found it, and what was the difference to him if he did get mixed up a little on his facts."[10]

The D.O.s could legitimately complain about his charge that they were "not engaged in critically building [osteopathy] up." The first school had been founded eighteen years earlier, with only four months of instruction given. Within six years, the D.O.s had established the Associated Colleges of Osteopathy (ACO) and the American Osteopathic Association (AOA), which set standards covering osteopathic schools and put into law minimum educational requirements for licensure. By 1898, the course was lengthened to two years (a total of twenty months) and in 1904, to three years (a total of twenty-seven months). At the time Flexner was conducting his survey, some of the schools were offering a fourth year of instruction. In addition, the AOA conducted its first evaluation survey of all osteopathic schools in 1903, three years before the AMA did likewise for M.D-granting institutions. This process of setting and upgrading standards may have helped stimulate a decline in the number of osteopathic colleges from thirteen in 1901 to eight at the time of Flexner's tour. From the D.O.s' point of view, this was real progress which Flexner did not bother to mention, or simply could not appreciate.[11] The AOA Board of Trustees declared.

We have no apologies for our colleges. They have done well, and we take pride in their attainments and in their ambitions and determinations to teach most thoroughly and scientifically all that pertains to disease in all its phases and manifestations. We demand they be allowed to do this, according to the needs of our profession and not in accord with the wishes of any self-appointed, self-seeking, tyrannical and prejudicial judges.[12]

Interestingly, the AOA's own Committee on Education in its annual reports had substantially agreed with Flexner on the problem of low entrance standards. Students were routinely admitted without high school diplomas. Also, the committee complained of poor basic science laboratories, lack of sufficient clinical facilities, an inadequate teaching corps. Although its own surveys had noted the same deficiencies that Flexner had documented, the committee's findings were not accompanied by Flexner's vitriolic prose. Unlike Flexner, who evaluated all schools with an ideal institution—Johns Hopkins—in mind, D.O. college inspectors were pragmatically oriented, recognizing the limited possibilities for amelioration under existing conditions. To them, reform was proceeding at a reasonable pace.[13]

THE NEXT TWENTY-FIVE YEARS

In the twenty-five years following the issuance of the "Flexner Report," several significant improvements in M.D. undergraduate education were made based on efforts underway before Flexner. Higher entrance standards were set and maintained. In 1914, the AMA CME mandated that all incoming medical students must have completed one year of college work. This was extended to two years in 1918. As of 1936, 83 percent of all matriculants exceeded this minimum and close to 50 percent enrolled with a baccalaureate degree.[14] The instructional program was greatly enhanced, largely because of changes in the surviving colleges' fiscal condition. During the 1934 to 1935 and 1935 to 1936 academic years, 55 percent of the total income of all accredited M.D.-granting schools was raised through taxes, public and private general university funds, and philanthropy.[15] With the additional revenue these sources brought, the colleges built more completely outfitted laboratories, hired full-time professors, and upgraded and expanded their hospital and dispensary facilities. In addition, commercial and otherwise weak schools closed for lack of students or were forced out of business. By 1935, the number of non-sectarian schools decreased from 107 to 64, a loss of 40 percent. M.D.-granting sectarian schools were hit much harder. The number of homeopathic schools dropped from fourteen to two (an 86 percent decline) and eclectic schools sank from eight to one (an 88 percent decrease). Osteopathic schools dropped only from eight to seven (12 percent).

During this same twenty-five year period, the D.O.s lagged far behind the M.D.s in the reform of their undergraduate educational system. With respect to pre-professional education, the AOA Board of Trustees stipulated in 1920 that each accredited college maintain an entrance standard of no less than a high school diploma. Yet no attempt was made to immediately enforce this provision, and it was not until the early 1930s that all schools appeared to fully comply.[16]

Those D.O.s in favor of stringent entrance standards were a decided minority. The Los Angeles college established a compulsory requirement of one year of college in 1920, but this was in response to a California law which mandated it. Most D.O.s sided with Dr. George Laughlin, who championed the "poor boy argument." Laughlin, who became head of the Kirksville school in the mid 1920s, argued that requiring two years of prior college work was hurting the underprivileged since they could least afford the additional schooling. As many of the students who did not meet this requirement came from farms and small towns, the standard had the indirect effect of causing a decline in the percentage of recent M.D. graduates deciding to locate in sparsely populated areas. Without this requirement, D.O. schools could meet the needs of the economically disadvantaged student and help alleviate the growing rural physician shortage. As it turned out, Laughlin's views and predictions had merit, since the D.O.s traditionally are highly represented in rural areas, and historically D.O. students have come from less affluent backgrounds than their M.D. counterparts.[17]

However, the main reason militating against a further increase in preprofessional requirements for D.O.s was the economic condition of the colleges themselves. Although the schools became non-profit institutions during this period, the sources of their funding remained unchanged. Unlike most M.D.-granting schools, they received no tax support, no general university monies, and comparatively little outside philanthropy. In 1932, reportedly 92 percent of the gross receipts of all the colleges were secured from tuition alone.[18] In other words, the schools' very survival depended on their ability to obtain a base number of new matriculants each fall. By setting the preprofessional standard at the M.D. level of two years of college or more, the osteopathic schools would be drastically cutting their pool of eligible applicants, and the quota of students necessary to meet expenses would very likely not be reached.

The educational program of the osteopathic schools, however, did undergo a number of important changes between 1910 and 1935. All the colleges added a mandatory fourth academic year in 1916, and after much debate and struggle the AOA finally approved a required standard course in materia medica and pharmacology for inclusion in the curriculum in 1929. As a result of these reforms, the profession would boast in its promotional literature that in terms of subjects presented and time devoted to them, M.D. and D.O. schools were equivalent. Indeed on paper osteopathic institutions offered students a few hundred more clock hours of training than the typical M.D.-granting school. However, this was a deceptive figure. Although the length of basic science courses in D.O. schools was greatly expanded, the instruction itself continued to be weak. Some preclinical teachers were now full-time, but these were D.O.s few of whom possessed graduate degrees in the subjects they taught. The equipment remained meager, and most laboratories contained only the barest necessities. Finally the courses were not as encompassing as those in M.D. colleges, partly because of the different preprofessional backgrounds of M.D. and D.O. matriculants. Osteopathic curricula, for example, included instruction in elementary biology and chemistry, which medical students had mastered before beginning their formal professional education.[19]

There were also severe problems in clinical training. While all of the schools were operating larger hospitals in the mid-1930s than previously, they were still quite small. Most M.D. colleges easily surpassed the minimum of 200 beds available for teaching purposes under guidelines set by the AMA. The six AOA-accredited schools averaged only eighty-eight beds. Thus, where a minimum of 2,000 clock hours were devoted to bedside and outpatient teaching at M.D.-granting institutions, an average of only 860 hours were spent at these six D.O. schools. In short, whatever improvements were made, the entire undergraduate osteopathic educational program in general badly trailed M.D. education. Yet osteopathic medicine survived.[20]

THE DEMISE OF M.D.-GRANTING SECTARIAN SCHOOLS

Why was it that so many sectarian M.D.-granting schools failed in the twenty-five years after Flexner's survey while almost all the osteopathic colleges he visited continued to function? What does all this tell us about the perceived agents of change, and their actual power? In examining this period of educational reform, it appears that the capacity of sectarian M.D. and D.O. schools to survive rested on how well they did in three areas: recognition of their educational standards by others, their economic solvency, and their ability to draw students. Performance in these areas was interrelated.

Though autonomous through most of the nineteenth century, homeopathy and eclecticism were losing the power to govern themselves by the early twentieth century. When licensure laws were passed beginning in the 1870s, many states granted these sects as well as regular medicine their own licensure boards. Thus, each group had the power to test its own candidates. However, by the beginning of the twentieth century, a number of states attempted to achieve greater standardization by eliminating this system and replacing it with the composite board approach. In the new system there was one board whose members were likely to proportionally represent physicians from competing groups practicing in the state. As the homeopaths and eclectics collectively constituted no more than 15 percent of the total physician population in the country at the turn of the century, this change put them at a serious disadvantage. To protect these minorities, the composite boards were not allowed to test candidates on matters relating to drug therapeutics, the area of difference among the groups. However, all regular, homeopathic, and eclectic candidates had to pass the same test in the basic sciences and in certain clinical subjects. Furthermore, many composite boards had the power to deny recognition to inferior schools. In the first few decades of the twentieth century, graduates of sectarian M.D. colleges were increasingly finding themselves unable to take licensure exams as composite boards toughened their standards.[21]

In 1904, the AMA created its CME. In 1906–07 its secretary, Dr. Nathan P. Colwell, inspected each M.D.-granting college then in operation with the goal of developing national requirements governing all undergraduate medical education. At the end of his visits, members of the AMA CME agreed to meet with members of the committees on education of The American Institute of Homeopathy and the National Confederation of Eclectic Medical Colleges at the latters' invitation to see if a common set of standards could be agreed upon by all three groups. Nothing apparently came of this. It is evident from the minutes of the meeting that the two sectarian organizations were afraid, quite appropriately, that the AMA CME was set on maintaining higher requirements for minimum undergraduate medical education than they were willing to impose upon their colleges.[22]

In 1910, the AMA CME released its first list of Class A or approved schools. Three years later, the CME indicated which colleges were in Class B: on probation, and in Class C: unacceptable. Meanwhile, composite boards were coming to the conclusion that therapeutic differences between regular medicine and the sects did not justify maintaining two separate standards governing medical education. If homeopathic and eclectic schools wanted recognition, they should be judged on an equal basis with non-sectarian institutions. The only on-going national program that existed to meet this need was the AMA classification system.

Marxist and other critics are correct in pointing out that orthodox medical reformers were in favor of the elimination of the homeopathic and eclectic systems. Certainly, all of the members of the CME as well as the secretary who was the major inspector were regular physicians, and shared Flexner's belief that "scientific medicine" knew no sectarian creed. However, the minutes of the CME, which include narrative summaries of inspections of sectarian schools, appear to be straightforward in their analyses. The CME's one-hundred-point scale used in evaluating all schools did not cover the content of courses pertaining to drug therapeutics, although the facilities for teaching pharmacology or homeopathic "drug provings" were fair game for evaluation.[23]

The initial ratings of homeopathic schools by the AMA compared reasonably well with orthodox medical colleges. Six of thirteen homeopathic institutions received Class A or acceptable ratings, compared to fifty-six of 111 non-sectarian degree-granting schools. On the other hand, eclectic schools were not viewed as satisfactory. None of the seven eclectic colleges received an A rating; and in 1913, when Class B and C ratings were first publicly differentiated, only one eclectic school even received a Class B.[24] Because state medical boards increasingly relied on AMA rankings to decide which medical schools should be recognized, a Class C and even a Class B ranking posed a real problem to sectarian as well as to regular schools.

Whether homeopathic and eclectic institutions could obtain or maintain Class A ranking depended less on the prejudices of AMA CME than on their ability to obtain large and continuing amounts of money to support their educational programs. Medical schools that could become integrated components of universities were in the best position to generate public and private funding to build new facilities, upgrade their equipment, provide greater laboratory and clinical training for students, and hire full-time faculty. Many regular medical schools could make such arrangements. Most sectarian schools could not. In 1910, only three sectarian colleges, all homeopathic, had ties to universities. The other eighteen sectarian M.D.-granting schools were thus at a distinct disadvantage. The great majority could depend only on revenues generated by tuition and this was not enough.

For sectarian schools to survive they needed to attract students, and in the case of homeopathy and eclecticism the proportion of students studying at these institutions had been declining for several decades. In 1880, homeopathic and eclectic students represented 17 percent of all medical students, in 1890—12 percent, in 1900—10 percent, in 1910— 6 percent, and in 1920—less than 4 percent.[25] In addition, homeopathic and eclectic schools had far fewer students per institution throughout this period. For example, in 1880, regular medical schools averaged 127 students, homeopathic schools averaged eighty-seven, and eclectic colleges averaged 103 students. Using Flexner's data, in 1909 non-sectarian schools averaged fifty-three more students than they had in 1880, homeopathic colleges nine less, and eclectic schools fifty-five less.[26]

For sectarian schools, all of which relied heavily on tuition, these declining numbers meant a decreasing amount of revenue available to improve, let alone maintain, existing facilities. This in turn meant a more difficult struggle for schools to secure approval from state licensure boards. Again using Flexner's 1909 data, the total income available per student based on tuition and other subsidies was $188 for regular schools, $102 for homeopathic colleges, and $91 for eclectic institutions. Overall, the total average income was $33,730 for regular M.D.-granting schools, $7,982 for homeopathic colleges, and $4,459 for eclectic institutions.[27] Clearly, homeopathic and eclectic medical educational programs were in financial trouble long before the CME and Flexner appeared.

Why were these sectarian schools unable to attract sufficient students? A chief reason seems to be that the distinctive philosophy and practices underlying these sectarian movements were rapidly fading. In the last quarter of the nineteenth century, homeopathic and eclectic physicians were coming closer to regular physicians in their conception of disease and in the therapies they employed. Furthermore, as Rothstein has argued, more students were choosing medical schools on the basis of perceived quality in facilities, equipment, and faculty. Thus, both regular and irregular weaker schools were losing out in this selection process. Some sectarian colleges responded by charging students less than regular schools and accepting students with lower credentials, but this did not bring enrollment figures to adequate levels. Even many alumni of sectarian schools were telling prospective medical students to go to regular colleges for a better education.[28]

Unable to secure approved status from state licensing boards, maintain economic solvency or attract students, most sectarian M.D. schools could not remain open. By 1935, there were only two homeopathic schools left, Hahnemann Medical College of Philadelphia and New York Homeopathic Medical College, non-university affiliated institutions that survived on the support of loyal alumni and local benefactors who could fund needed improvements to keep up with rising AMA requirements. Chicago Homeopathic, which had received a Class A rating in 1910, was unable to generate sufficient funds. Consequently its rating was lowered, it lost students, and by the mid–1920s ceased to exist.[29] Three university-affiliated homeopathic schools that shared facilities with regular medical colleges at the University of Michigan, University of Iowa, and Ohio State were closed in large part for lack of students.[30] Boston University Medical College dropped its homeopathic identity in 1918, seeing this change to be in the school's best interest, while the other schools closed relatively quickly after 1910. In 1935, the AMA told Hahnemann and New York Medical College that they would no longer inspect "sectarian" schools; consequently both dropped their homeopathic identity, which by then was mostly nominal.[31]

Between 1910 and 1920, the number of eclectic schools had dropped from eight to one, the sole survivor being the Eclectic Medical Institute of Cinncinati established in 1845. For a time, the institute struggled along with a Class B ranking; ultimately it sank to Class C status. Few states other than Ohio would recognize its graduates. Lack of support from its alumni and failure to attract students finally caused this last educational vestige of eclecticism to close its doors in 1939.[32] Both homeopathy and eclecticism lost the power to regulate themselves. They could not raise sufficient capital to maintain minimally acceptable, externally set educational standards, nor were they able to attract students. In contrast, osteopathic medicine during this period did relatively well in all three areas.

REASONS FOR THE SURVIVAL OF OSTEOPATHIC SCHOOLS

While most sectarian M.D.-granting colleges closed between 1910 and 1935, the number of osteopathic schools decreased by only one. Why did these institutions survive? Because their schools did not originally teach pharmacology, D.O.s were able to convince legislators and judges that, legally speaking, osteopathy was not the practice of medicine. They were also able to obtain separate licensing laws governing their practice.

By 1923, of forty-six states that had passed such legislation, twenty-seven had given D.O.s independent boards. Even in many of the states where D.O.s were examined for licensure by a composite board, the law generally specified minimum educational requirements that were lower for D.O.s and accepted a school's accreditation by the AOA as the sole criterion for a candidate's eligibility. Thus, osteopathy had won a considerable degree of autonomy.[33]

Unlike the AMA which was strongly committed to both dramatically raising standards and dramatically reducing the number of schools and graduates, the AOA was principally concerned with maintaining its existing number of schools and insuring an adequate enrollment, thus encouraging change at a pace schools could accommodate. This latter policy was not seriously challenged by legislators for many years, for they continued to view osteopathic colleges as different from medical schools, in large part because of the difference in degrees awarded. They essentially agreed with the osteopaths that the latter, unlike the homeopaths and the eclectics, did not have to meet the same standards for recognition and approval.

D.O. schools were attracting an adequate supply of students. In 1909, according to Flexner's figures, the average number of students per osteopathic school was 168, only 7 percent smaller than non-sectarian M.D. colleges. By 1926, the approximate average number of students per osteopathic school had risen to 255, just 6 percent smaller than the average for regular M.D.-granting colleges.[34]

As previously noted, osteopathic schools continued to be almost completely dependent upon tuition as their source of revenue. As long as the AOA did not require them to make major reforms, this situation did not cause serious difficulties. Since at the time of the "Flexner Report," osteopathic institutions were charging relatively high tuition, the revenue generated per student was not significantly lower than the average for all regular M.D. schools, although 25 percent of the latter were receiving funds from sources other than tuition. The D.O. colleges averaged $151 per student, $37 less than regular schools but $48 more than homeopathic ones and $60 more than the average for eclectic colleges. The total average income for D.O. schools in 1909 was $25,394; $8,336 less than regular M.D.-granting institutions, but $17,412 more than homeopathic and $20,935 more than eclectic colleges.[35] Clearly, D.O. schools were in a better economic position than other sectarian institutions.

During this period, as M.D. schools were requiring two or more years of undergraduate credits and many D.O. colleges were not even completely enforcing the high school graduation requirement, osteopathic institutions could appeal to students who wanted to become physicians but did not have the grades or pre-professional credits to get into an

M.D. school, regular or sectarian. Nevertheless, more students seem to have been attracted to osteopathy because of its methods than its low standards. The distinctive aspects of homeopathy and eclecticism were being de-emphasized by sectarian M.D. colleges. Prospective students generally saw them as reflecting "old-fashioned" or metaphysical thinking. However, osteopathy's emphasis upon physically manipulating structure to alter function probably seemed more materialistic and capable of achieving significant results. Indeed, in stressing their distinctive philosophy and degree as the real alternative to regular medicine, osteopathic schools lured students who might otherwise have chosen the colleges of other sects.

ACCELERATED CHANGE IN OSTEOPATHIC EDUCATION

Given their success at maintaining their autonomy, economic solvency, and student supply in the first third of this century, osteopathy might well have continued at the same relatively slow pace of reform. However, changes in the D.O.s' scope of practice made this increasingly difficult. By the mid 1920s, D.O.s were widely viewed as "entering medicine through the back door."[36] While in some states D.O.s could be legally recognized as "physicians and surgeons" eligible for the same unlimited license as M.D.s, in many others they were blocked by legislation. Legislators agreed with the state medical societies' position that, if the D.O.s wanted to be licensed as complete physicians and surgeons, they needed to meet the same basic educational standards M.D.s met. By the mid 1930s, some lawmakers in unlimited-license states were in favor of commissioning independent investigations of osteopathic undergraduate education with an eye to possibly revoking their existing privileges, particularly after a survey of D.O. schools by two Canadian M.D. educators indicated a wide gap in standards between M.D. and D.O. schools.[37] Furthermore, the inferiority of the osteopathic educational program was reflected in poor results in medical and composite licensure board examinations, as well as in basic science board tests required in several states that had separate M.D. and D.O. boards.[38]

If D.O. graduates could not become licensed to practice in the state they chose, or could not practice the full measure of what they had been taught in college, before long the schools would not attract enough students. This, in turn, would directly affect their economic solvency. With the survival of their movement threatened by the legislatures and the state boards, reformers within the profession convinced the colleges and the AOA that they had no choice but to make fundamental changes in the structure and quality of their educational system.

In retrospect, the transformation of osteopathic colleges in the second quarter-century following the "Flexner Report" (from 1935 to 1960) constitutes an achievement no less remarkable than that accomplished by the M.D.s in the first quarter-century, particularly as it occurred without the benefits of tax, university, or outside philanthropic support. Despite the knowledge that enrollment would suffer, the AOA mandated a one-year college prerequisite in 1938, and adopted the two-year standard in 1940. As a result, enrollment declined 21 percent between 1937 and 1940. This drop was accelerated by America's entry into World War II, when the schools' enrollment declined to about 25 percent of the pre-hostilities level. One osteopathic school which had long been struggling closed, leaving six. After the war, an active recruitment effort focused at undergraduate colleges resulted in an influx of new students. By 1947, enrollment had returned to the level it had reached before the introduction of the two-year college requirement, and the ratio of applicants to available places in osteopathic schools rose to two to one, thus making possible the selection of better-qualified students. By 1954, all osteopathic colleges had set a three-year college prerequisite, and by 1960, 71 percent of all new osteopathic matriculants had a baccalaureate or advanced degree.[39]

The content and orientation of the curriculum also changed. New basic science facilities were built, and students spent approximately 60 percent of their time in the laboratory as opposed to the lecture hall during the first two years. D.O.s who had traditionally taught the basic sciences were increasingly being replaced in many fields by full-time Ph.D.s. On the clinical side, actual bedside and outpatient experience for each student was almost tripled by 1960, because the colleges expanded their own hospitals and forged new arrangements for clinical instruction with other osteopathic facilities.[40]

Many of these changes in undergraduate osteopathic medical education were made possible because the schools placed themselves in a more secure economic position. In 1943, when enrollment had sunk to an all-time low, the AOA established what eventually became known as the Osteopathic Progress Fund. Practitioners in the field were solicited for contributions, and many rallied to the colleges' support. This money, which amounted to millions of dollars, was directly channeled into college treasuries. This allowed the schools not only to survive, but to upgrade themselves. The period also marked the beginning of federal support, as D.O.s won the right to receive Public Health Service training grants and their schools received Hill-Burton construction funds.[41]

There were significant advances on the post-doctoral level as well. In 1936, the AOA Bureau of Hospitals undertook its first inspection of institutions offering internships. Since the primary objective of the association was to provide a position for every new graduate, requirements were set low to qualify as many hospitals as possible. During World War II, the D.O.s, exempt from the draft and ineligible for service with the military medical corps, began taking care of the clients of inducted M.D.s. Since regular hospitals refused the osteopaths admitting and staff privileges, their new patients helped underwrite the costs of building and maintaining private osteopathic institutions. In 1945, there were approximately 260 osteopathic hospitals, more than triple the number of a decade earlier. This in turn helped alleviate the internship shortage, and by 1951 available positions surpassed the number of that year's graduating seniors, thus making possible the toughening of program standards. A similar development was taking place with respect to residency programs.[42]

The push for higher standards between 1935 and 1960 resulted in progress on the legal front. At the end of this time, D.O.s were eligible for unlimited licensure in thirty-eight states. Osteopathic schools were now able to meet the requirements of certain medical boards and other governmental agencies newly empowered to approve them, and D.O. graduates possessed a pre-professional background and postgraduate training matching or exceeding the minimum called for by each state. Osteopathic performance on outside examinations also showed significant gains. Although from 1942 to 1953 results obtained by M.D.s on basic science board tests remained virtually unchanged (86–87 percent pass), the D.O.s went from 52 percent pass to 80 percent pass. Significant improvements were made by D.O.s before state medical and composite boards of licensure. Where the results of U.S. medical graduates remained constant at 96 percent pass from 1940 to 1959, the D.O.s climbed from 62 percent pass total to 81 percent—still behind, but clearly closing the gap. By the early 1970s, the percentage of D.O.s passing such exams was no different from the percentage of M.D.s.[43]

By 1960 there were still critical problems that D.O. schools needed to solve, but there was no doubt that they had placed their educational program upon a more solid foundation. In the third twenty-five year period following the "Flexner Report" (1960 to 1985), the D.O.s, assisted by an infusion of new funding, would continue to make significant strides to improve and expand their educational program.[44]

The "Flexner Report" did help to accelerate changes in medical education in the early part of this century, but the standardization of the system was due first of all to the AMA, which could use the report to further its own goals. The AMA wanted to dramatically raise requirements and at the same time reduce the number of graduates. Homeopathic and eclectic national organizations wanted to do neither but could not maintain control over the accreditation of their educational programs. The state medical boards had the ultimate say over the recognition of schools, and most used the AMA ratings as their guide. As the great majority of sectarian M.D. colleges could not obtain sufficient funds to upgrade their institutions, attract an adequate supply of students, and obtain approved status, they had to close. On the other hand, those viable homeopathic schools which did well on all three criteria were eventually pressured by the AMA to drop their sectarian identity. In contrast, the AOA both before and after the "Flexner Report" maintained its control over the accreditation of osteopathic colleges and set its standards governing approval relatively low in order to keep schools operating. Unlike the homeopathic and eclectic colleges, tuition alone supported the schools. Only when the AOA's power was threatened by state legislatures and the state medical and composite boards of licensure—because its schools' teachings and its practitioners' scope of practice expanded—did it significantly reform the educational system. In this it was successful. As a result, state boards would continue to recognize AOA accreditation ratings in approving osteopathic schools. This autonomy, along with the schools' continuing ability to attract students and maintain economic solvency, largely explains why the fate of osteopathic undergraduate medical education was different from that of its homeopathic and eclectic counterparts.

7

American Health Services Since the "Flexner Report"

Odin W. Anderson

The current American health services delivery system appears fragmented, uncoordinated, unplanned, and untidy to those who carry their own rational models in their heads. If, however, we review carefully the development of this infrastructure over the last one hundred years it has a logic of its own stemming from the characteristics of the liberal-democratic political process and the relatively open and mixed economy.

I have divided the development of the American health services into three periods.[1] During the first, from 1875 to 1930, the basic infrastructure of the health care system was created. The second period, from 1930 to 1965, was characterized by the emergence of third-party reimbursement. In the third period, which began in 1965 and will extend indefinitely into the future, we have the creation of mechanisms to manage and control a health care system that is perceived to have gotten out of control.

THE DEVELOPMENT OF THE INFRASTRUCTURE, 1875 TO 1930

In this initial period, the private fee-for-service practice of medicine was the norm, as were private non-profit sectarian and community hospitals with voluntary citizen boards. Initially surgeons, then other types of physicians, reached agreements with the hospitals to admit their private patients; in return the doctors provided charity care for poor, non-paying patients. The hospitals were then able to maintain their non-profit, tax-exempt status as institutions dispensing charity. An emerging and broad segment of the population with a discretionary income unlike anything in contemporary Europe appeared in America after the Civil War as a product of the tremendous economic and industrial expansion in the country. This enabled the growth of a health services infrastructure which was privately owned and operated. The growing middle income group supported this structure, in the main on a pay-as-you-go basis. The hospitals received their building capital from wealthy philanthropists and community fund drives. No other country has been able to achieve this magnitude of private support, which became the backbone of the health services delivery system.[2]

During this period the country was in the political heyday of limited government support, except for the public school system and subsidies to the railroads through grants of land. Private philanthropy and very grudging state and local support from tax sources helped to pay for the care of the poor. In fact personal health services were regarded as an individual problem to be paid for like any other commodity or service. Such things as clean water, clean milk, clean streets, and immunization were felt to be legitimate public problems.

It is significant that Flexner was not interested in the system behind the delivery of personal health services. He, like others through the era of voluntary health insurance and Medicare and Medicaid, accepted as a given that the free-standing physician or physician group and the free-standing hospital both charged fees.

It was an individualistic age that emphasized the quality of the individual, and, in the case of medical reformers such as Flexner and the AMA, the quality of the individual doctor. Flexner and his many like-minded contemporaries were interested in abolishing mediocrity.[3] The quality of the individual doctor was to be improved by improving the quality of the medical school, even if this resulted in closing many of them. Licenses were to be provided only to those physicians who were products of acceptable medical schools, thus eliminating both unfit schools and unfit physicians. Flexner was not worried about reducing the absolute number of doctors, since poorly trained physicians were no use. He did believe, however, that there would be enough doctors after the reforms were made.[4]

In any case, the American people supported this infrastructure growth, and the number of hospitals and hospital beds, specialization, and the use of health services all continued to increase. By 1930, an infrastructure had developed whose characteristics are with us today, currently undergoing structural transformation, but still essentially privately owned. We continue to have the municipal public hospitals as functional spillovers for the private non-profit hospitals. The investor-owned hospitals had a resurgence after their relative diminution in the 1920s, but are now probably stabilizing as a worrisome minority to the non-profit hospitals. The poor continue to be treated as a class in terms of access.[5]

It appears that Flexner and others were pleased with the improved quality of physicians by the 1930s. The medical school and delivery structures were in place and momentum toward quality was maintained. Emphasis on science and research led to specialization and complicated surgery. These in turn led to higher costs for both training and delivery, and further led to the reduction in the number of physicians in rural areas and inner cities. And as the episodes of costly illnesses increased, health insurance was devised to protect families from these contingencies.

THE ERA OF THIRD-PARTY REIMBURSEMENT, 1930 TO 1965

Of course, historical stages overlap, so it is necessary to backtrack to trace the events that led to widespread acceptance of third-party payment for health services. While the infrastructure was taking shape and the quality of physicians and medical schools were improving, another problem began to get serious attention. Little was known about how the general public used the imposing health services edifice that had been created, how that use was paid for, and what the needs of the public were, as measured by morbidity and mortality patterns. Further, it seemed reasonable to examine the structure and operation of the mainstream delivery system and also to study other emerging delivery systems, such as group practice with prepayment and other health insurance arrangements. The vehicle for this examination was the Committee on the Costs of Medical Care (CCMC), organized with a fund of about one million dollars from six foundations.

The creation of the CCMC was stimulated, it seems, by the failure to inaugurate universal health insurance. Popular political support for this was lacking, even among labor unions. The advocates of universal health insurance were primarily public health physicians, economists who were products of the Progressive Era, social workers, a few academic physicians, and health statisticians. The main coordinating agency was the American Association for Labor Legislation. Supporters of health insurance after World War I sponsored a massive research effort into need and demand for health services and new types of delivery systems, such as group practice. They believed in the power of facts to induce social reform, feeling that information would transcend political pressure groups. Many of the original group, plus a new cadre of relatively young experts, staffed the CCMC studies. Conspicuous among them was Michael M. Davis, a sociologist who began to promote some form of government health insurance. Also prominent among the staff was C. Rufus Rorem, an economist, who later promoted a form of voluntary health insurance which became the Blue Cross Hospital Plan.[6]

Among the twenty-eight published reports of the CCMC, the most significant document was a survey of the use of and expenditures for personal health services of a large sample of the American population, including morbidity patterns.[7] This study was the first of its kind in the world.

Early in this period there was little concern with physician quality as a separate variable; instead attention focused on public access to care, which was assumed to be of acceptable quality. In fact, R. I. Lee and L. W. Jones were bold enough to formulate need/demand norms based on the morbidity patterns in the survey.[8] They estimated the appropriate rates for utilization of physician, dentist, and hospital services in relation to need. Not surprisingly, they found that effective demand was appreciably below the authors' norm of need. Their effort was the first (and last) attempt to estimate need and appropriate use and supply in a systematic fashion. Why was it the last attempt? I would speculate that the many CCMC reports, especially the document on which Lee and Jones based their estimates, were used for a long time as basic sources of data for health policy formulation. There may have been no felt need for further studies. Also, during and after World War II, use of services was increasing, which was a major policy objective for the country; so studies of the relationship between need and demand seemed unnecessary. Finally, as epidemiologists, sociologists, and economists became much more sophisticated in this type of research methodology, they were unwilling to be as bold as Lee and Jones.

One initiative, with its beginnings in the previous period, was aimed at improving the standards of hospitals. In 1918, the American College of Surgeons began to survey hospitals as to their suitability for performing surgical operations. It studied 692 institutions with more than one-hundred beds, and only 12.9 percent were approved. By 1933, 1,603 hospitals with more than one-hundred beds were surveyed and 93.9 percent were approved.[9] As more and more specialties were established, concerns with the overall quality of the hospital became pervasive. The result was the creation in 1951 of the Joint Commission on Accreditation of Hospitals, which included representation from the American College of Surgeons, the American College of Physicians, the American Hospital Association, and the AMA. The criteria to evaluate hospitals expanded considerably, but continued to relate mainly to structure and process rather than outcome: board certification and experience of surgeons, access to equipment and personnel as determined by medical and surgical specialists, and the practice of postmortems and clinical-pathological conferences. Very prominent were criteria for building standards, such as the width of corridors and doors for personnel traffic, ambulatory beds, and wheel chairs; the absence of fire hazards; and cleanliness. The pervasive drive was for higher and higher standards as ends in themselves.

A supporting aspect of the thrust toward hospital quality was the professionalization of hospital administration through certification and education. In this initiative, Michael M. Davis is Abraham Flexner's counterpart. Davis wanted to make hospital administration a learned profession like medicine.[10] As a private consultant and as an officer of the Julius Rosenwald Foundation, Davis surveyed hospitals and clinics. During the 1920s and early 1930s he traveled through every state in the union and had the opportunity to visit hospitals of all sizes, consulting with many administrators, trustees, and medical staff members. He concluded that the administrators were too absorbed in daily details and they lacked skills in human relations and standard business practices. A professionally trained hospital administrator should know how to manage a hospital with due consideration for the needs of physicians to practice at their optimum and for the general needs of patient comfort and care. The administrator was the custodian of the institutional resources and the physician was the patient's advocate. The professional administrator should be able to integrate these two roles. An elite group of hospital administrators supported this effort to upgrade their profession. In 1933, leading hospital administrators established the American College of Hospital Administrators (now called the American College of Health Care Executives), emulating the American College of Surgeons.

With a grant from the Julius Rosenwald Foundation, in 1934 Davis established the first graduate program in hospital administration in the country, as well as in the world, at the Graduate School of Business, University of Chicago. He originally wanted at least two physician trainees a year, but could not fill this quota.

Since 1945 there has been a rapid expansion of graduate programs in health services administration (this new term replaced hospital administration as the occupational niches broadened). The Kellogg Foundation provided startup money for many of these. There are now about sixty programs in the United States with more than 5,000 students and about 1,500 graduates per year.[11] Thus, hospital administrators have become trained professionals with appropriate degrees. A minority are physicians.

During this period, there was a planned increase in the numbers of both health care institutions and personnel. In 1946 the Hospital Survey and Construction Act was passed with the goal of providing start-up capital for hospital construction, particularly in rural areas. In the 1950s and 1960s there was federal contribution in one form or another to increase the supply of physicians, nurses, and supporting personnel, based on the consensus that there was a shortage. All through this period quality of services, was not an issue. There seemed to be a feeling that, in general, quality was good, but that improvements could be made. A momentum seemed to assure positive change. General indicators were used as surrogates for quality, such as the number of board-certified physicians and the fact that physicians had been trained in university-based medical schools with elaborate research programs.[12]

While all these developments were taking place concurrently, the major force increasing access to services was the third-party private (voluntary) health insurance and later in 1965 the federal Medicare Act for the elderly and the federal-state Medicaid Act for the poor. Medicare and Medicaid came late in the third-party era; by this time 75 to 80 percent of the population was covered by private insurance. This broad coverage was the result, in large part, of labor-management negotiations for health insurance as a fringe benefit. The third party made access to health services easier by abolishing, or at least reducing, the cost to patients at time of service.

The great expansion in health insurance made cost much less visible to patients at the time of service and freed physicians from the previous cost-consciousness they felt when patients did not have insurance. This led to allegations of over-use of services, encouraged by the fee-for-service method of reimbursement. It is generally assumed that this method of paying physicians creates an incentive to recommend more units of service than necessary, and naturally has implications for quality as well. "Necessary" is very difficult to define in operation except for practices that are obviously gross and relatively infrequent. A pioneering attempt to monitor physician practice patterns in a medical prepayment arrangement was tried in 1937 by researchers at the School of Public Health at the University of Michigan. The research took place in a prepaid plan in Windsor, Ontario, which offered home and office calls as well as in-patient physicians' service.[13] The method analyzed physicians' practice patterns to isolate outliers who appeared to be ordering more visits and laboratory work than the majority of physicians. The objective of the method was to control volume and, therefore, costs, but it also had quality implications if one assumes that more was not necessarily better. The same method was used in the physician prepayment plans sponsored by the county medical societies in the State of Washington. These Medical Bureaus are still in existence.

Another attempt to evaluate medical practice was made in North Carolina by researchers at the University of North Carolina who studied the practice patterns of a sample of private general practitioners.[14] They concluded that 40 percent of their sample were practicing mediocre or bad medicine by what the investigators regarded as standard professional criteria. The study evoked a great deal of interest and concern but has not been repeated, except in Canada where the investigator used the same methods.[15] The implications of these results for medical education were that general practice and general internal medicine should have longer and more rigorous training in order to inculcate standards of care that would be maintained even under difficult circumstances.

Another attempt at measuring quality indirectly was made in the mid–1950s as a spinoff from a series of national surveys of households as to their use of and expenditures for health services. This study was modeled more or less on the CCMC survey of 1928 to 1931.[16] Utilizing the prevailing assumption that board certification should result in higher quality physician performance, national household surveys in 1953, 1958, and 1963 collected data on the proportion of inpatient surgical procedures performed by board-certified surgeons. In 1953, 37 percent of all hospital-based surgery was performed by board certified surgeons; in 1958, it was 40 percent; and in 1963, it was 46 percent.

A small cloud on the horizon was the emergence of group practice prepayment plans as a spinoff of the group practice concept. This development was regarded as a threat (which it was) to the mainstream solo practice, fee-for-service arrangement in that physicians were on a salary in contract with a plan. A plan had a known group of physicians, a known population to be served, a known number of hospital beds, a known range of services to be provided, and a known annual budget. Plans were under one overall management. The proponents of group practice with prepayment claimed that it assured high quality, appropriate medical judgment and services in one place, and an emphasis on preventive services. Prepared plans have come to be called Health Maintenance Organizations (HMOs). The original and continuing motive was to provide good quality and convenient service at a reasonable, not necessarily low, cost.[17] It was (and is) assumed that with the power to select physicians for a proper mix of specialties and the presumption that these physicians would more likely act as a team in monitoring medical standards, the quality would in general be higher than that prevailing in the mainstream fee-for-service arrangement. I allude to this development because Flexner appears not to have conceived of the influence of the structure of health services delivery on the practice styles of physicians. Nor do medical schools even today deal in any substance with this issue. Quality concepts and standards began to be introduced into delivery systems, on the understanding that even with generally high quality medical schools, physicians vary considerable in their practice patterns.

THE ERA OF MANAGEMENT AND CONTROL, 1965 TO THE FUTURE

After the Medicare and Medicaid programs went into operation in 1966, following the legislation authorizing them the previous year, about 85 percent of the population was covered by one form of insurance or another. The mainstream organizational structure of the delivery system and its method of paying providers—retrospective reimbursement based on charges and/or costs—assured little incentive for hospitals and physicians to watch costs closely. In retrospect this open-ended method of funding seems irresponsible, but the whole economy was irresponsible in a period of tremendous economic expansion and increased personal income. Health services began to get both public- and private-sector attention when their prices rose faster than the general consumer price index. By the late 1960s this financing cornucopia aroused increasing concern about how to control the cost escalation. Again, quality as such was not questioned, but eventually concern with costs would implicate the quality of services.

The first political and official sign of the concern with costs was a mandate in the Medicare Act to monitor length of stay in the hospital. There was to be utilization review for Medicare patients by a committee of physicians in each hospital. Congress feared that utilization of services was an area with potential for abuse and thus chose to address directly the issue of physician decision-making. Utilization review (UR) was actually a fiscal control, but it was also rationalized as a quality control in that it was not good care to keep patients in the hospital longer than necessary. In any case, UR, began as a very small cloud on the horizon. When this method did not seem to have much effect on total days of care for Medicare patients, a more comprehensive process involving Professional Standards Review Organizations (PSROs) was introduced in 1972. At first, the AMA opposed UR, then accepted it in order to have more control. Two hundred or so PSRO areas were established in the country and hospitals were grouped within them to make comparisons more effective. The PSRO committees were made up exclusively of physicians. Again, the PSRO method did not contain costs satisfactorily, according to Congress.[18] In 1983 a much more stringent and detailed method called the Medicare Prospective Payment System (PPS) was inaugurated. Perversely, Congress never set a standard of reasonable cost. The fiscal control in the PPS is in the form of a budget cap on the diagnosis-related groups (DRGs). Based on national average of the costs of treating Medicare patients, the Health Care Financing Administration (HCFA) set a reimbursement limit on each DRG to make the hospitals (and physicians) cost-conscious. If hospitals exceeded the DRG reimbursement limit they lost money; if they were under the limit they kept the money. The DRG system is still "shaking down" operationally, and the ultimate consequence to hospitals, patients, and medical practice has not been determined. Quality issues are being raised by allegations of "premature" discharge.

It is therefore clear that this country is now in the period of managing and controlling the operation of the health services delivery system, a period which will never end. Physicians are now being managed more and more as part of a total system through fiscal controls and monitoring of practice patterns to identify seeming deviations from professional norms established by custom, precepts, art, and science. The primary method is control through fiscal incentives, the primary vehicle for the government being the DRG system. There appears to be a prevailing view that there is a lot of "fat" in the health care system and fiscal controls and incentives will squeeze it out, forcing the providers—particularly physicians—to relate costs of procedures to their efficacy.[19] However, there is, so far, no overall methodology to do so. It is hoped that variations in practice patterns will be narrowed, for the differences seem excessively large. The rate of hospital admissions and average length of stay vary widely for seemingly similar medical conditions. The rates of performance of certain surgical procedures also vary widely. Differences are to be expected, but researchers wonder if the range of these variations make medical sense. The extremes, they feel, must mean questionable quality of care.[20] There are, however, except for very gross practices, few systematically determined criteria to make judgments about appropriate levels of utilization.[21]

Payers are increasingly employing other controls on volume of use, controls with their own quality implications. These include screening the appropriateness of hospital admissions (in addition to length of stay) and encouraging or requiring a second opinion for surgery, strategies which are supposed to reduce unnecessary admissions and surgical procedures.

Academicians have begun to inaugurate research into the concepts and methods of controlling quality. The "blunderbuss" methods being used need a great deal of refinement and are far from perfected yet. Donabedian is the most noted conceptualizer,[22] another is Greene.[23] A critique of the current state of quality control was attempted by Anderson and Shields.[24] They argued that a generic method of volume and quality control of physicians' services should include setting up the appropriate organizational arrangement to change physicians' practice styles by competition between groups of physicians within known budgets, and not by direct intervention in physician decision-making as in PSROs and DRGs.

A recent crude and a desperate attempt to influence the quality of hospitals was the publication of figures released by HCFA of the death rates in hospitals serving Medicare patients. The public in effect was warned to stay away from comparatively high-death-rate hospitals, not correcting for case mix, severity of diagnosis, and complexities of surgical procedures.

Interestingly, in a 1983 survey of a national sample of 207 selected informants from medicine, insurance, politics, government, and labor, 57 percent believed the American health services were functioning "very well" and 36 percent "pretty well," adding up to a resounding 93 percent. On the other hand, however, 64 percent felt the system was functioning "very poorly" and 26 percent "pretty poorly" on containing costs, a total of 90 percent. This elite group of informants did not appear to equate high quality with high cost.[25] The inference is that quality can be maintained and improved at less expense.

OBSERVATIONS, PROJECTIONS, AND CONCLUSIONS

If Flexner were to rise from his grave today what would he say about what science and medical technology have wrought, some of the groundwork for which he and his contemporaries laid? Would he say there is too much specialization, too much medical reductionism, too much high technology, even though these are the direct results of his efforts and objectives? What would he say about the emerging proliferation of cost controls and their effects on quality? Would he advocate an expansion of primary care? Would he feel that the legitimate autonomy of physician decision-making is being eroded and that he did not intend that individualistic physicians should be herded into groups and have professional managers negotiate salaries, equipment, productivity, and other characteristics of the business-industrial model?

Until expenditures and prices for personal health services began to rise faster than the gross national product, the general public was encouraged to "see the doctor early." The increase in use of services was regarded as an end in itself. Indeed the proportion of the population who sought physician-services at least once in a year for any reason rose from 40 percent in the early 1930s to 75 percent in the mid–1980s. The rate of use of standard preventive services had also risen greatly. The view now is that the physician should be seen early, not as early as seems common, but just at the "right time." Now there is interest in determining the appropriate fit between need/demand and the personal health services infrastructure. Associated with this is the increasing concern with determining and implementing the proper specialty distribution of physicians, since there is a prevailing belief that there are too many specialists, particularly surgeons, and too few primary care practitioners.[26] Obviously, the present presumed maldistribution across specialties is a direct product of Flexner's mission to put medicine on as scientific a basis as possible. Is there now, however, a rational way to determine the proper mix in the delivery system? Such knowledge could guide medical schools in developing appropriate training programs. Are medical schools inherently able to serve this function or is it a responsibility of aspiring medical students to know the market and select specialties accordingly? Group practices and HMOs will be determining the proper mix for their own personnel through trial and error by measuring need/demand and referral patterns from generalists to specialists. Still, the powerful forces of science and technology will likely influence the mix of specialties, as medical reductionism to isolate disease entities for both diagnostic and therapeutic purposes is highly regarded clinically.

Will the medical profession be losing the autonomy that it gained during the period of the establishment of the health services infra-structure?[27] My own view is that physicians will not have the same free-dom as previously to determine the amount and method of payment and the overall characteristics of the delivery system but will continue in essence to have discretionary control over diagnoses and treatment. The current onslaught of DRGs and other methods to influence phy-sician decision-making will slow as the profession regroups to maintain standards. Already there are conferences being held on the possible impact of cost control on quality, one of which I helped organize.[28]

In support of this view I wish to paraphrase and quote at length the observations of a wise sociologist and colleague, W. R. Scott. He observes that it takes the creation of social and organizational structure to provide goals and motivation for participants in a system. So, in order to bring about desired change, one must create new structures. In hospitals or HMOs create the position of chief of professional services who is em-powered to negotiate rewards and penalties. Simply trying to exhort and persuade people on an individual basis to change their behavior will not work as well.

But then he warns that one should

never underestimate the inventiveness and the cussedness of individual mem-bers, particularly of work groups to redefine, to change, and to use these struc-tures to serve their own ends. Consequently, the search for some kind of absolute perfection in structure is always going to be an illusory search. We are going to create structures, and these structures are going to have both intended and unintended effects, and we are going to have to create new structures to deal with those unintended effects and so on. We really need to keep in mind both of these inevitable kinds of processes.[29]

Thus the 1990s will demand continuing attention and adaptation to paradoxes inherent in the complex enterprise called personal health services. One of the paradoxes is the observation I once heard that the personal physician is both indispensable and outmoded.

8

Trends in the Financing of Undergraduate Medical Education

Janet D. Perloff

After several decades of substantial federal subsidy, the financial base of undergraduate medical education is currently undergoing significant change. Federal support for medical education is being reduced and the costs of medical education are being shifted elsewhere, especially to the medical schools and to medical students. This chapter traces trends in medical education financing between 1950 and the present.

The first two sections describe and consider the implications of the phenomenal growth in federal support for biomedical research during the 1950s and the subsequent decline of this base of support during the 1960s. In the third and fourth sections, the period of direct federal support for medical education during the 1960s and 1970s is described. Finally, in the fifth and sixth sections, the gradual and continuing increase in medical school clinical revenues is documented. Adaptations made by medical schools to the shifting and sometimes precarious bases of their financial support are identified and implications of these adaptations for undergraduate medical education are considered.

The most significant adaptation medical schools have made to recently declining federal financial support has been increasing their reliance on the revenue generated by the clinical activities of faculty. In addition, some medical schools have found it necessary to increase their tuition and fees. Analysis of these shifting bases of support for medical education leads to the conclusion that medical schools presently face several critical challenges. The first is the need for medical schools to ensure the continued evolution of well-managed faculty practice plans which can attract patients in an increasingly competitive health care environment. The second is the need for medical schools to harness the resources of faculty practice plans in serving (or at least not ignoring) the best interests of medical education, medical students, and the surrounding community. The third is the need for medical schools to preserve equitable access to a medical education regardless of the student's ability to pay.

TRENDS IN FEDERAL BIOMEDICAL RESEARCH FUNDING

During the decades following publication of the "Flexner Report," the facilities and faculties of American medical schools gradually came under increasing strain. Rapid industrialization, urbanization, and population growth characterized the years following World War II. By the late 1940s there was a widely shared perception that new sources of revenue would be needed if American medical schools were to keep pace with the growing demand for the services of the medical profession.

The private sector was first to respond to the growing need to revitalize American medical schools and to increase the supply of physicians. The National Fund for Medical Education was established in 1949, mobilizing the financial resources of labor, corporations, professional organizations, foundations, and individuals. In addition, the Ford Foundation, the Commonwealth Fund, and other private foundations began to increase their support for medical education during this period.[1]

Direct federal support for medical education was repeatedly proposed during the late 1940s and early 1950s but the medical profession thwarted its enactment. Proposals introduced in Congress included provisions for capitation and construction grants for new and existing medical schools, as well as for scholarship support for medical students.[2] These proposals for direct federal support for medical education were vigorously opposed by the medical profession, which sought to preserve the autonomy of medical schools and "the freedom to describe, to choose, to regulate new entrants to the profession."[3]

The medical profession's opposition to direct federal support for medical education continued throughout the 1950s. At the same time, the AMA, the AAMC, and other organized interests fostered the congressional inclination to invest in biomedical research. Further incentive was provided by the Steelman Report of 1947, the Surgeon General's Committee on Medical School Grants and Finances of 1951, and the President's Commission on the Health Needs of the Nation of 1953, all of which advocated increasing the role of medical schools in conducting the nation's biomedical research.[4] At first, federal support was limited to biomedical research grants to medical faculty members, made primarily through the National Institutes of Health (NIH). In 1956, with the passage of the Health Facilities Research Act, support broadened to include the costs of constructing new facilities for federally sponsored research programs of medical school faculty. Concern was expressed over the evolving relationship between the government and universities and the potential for government interference in medical education.

However, federal support for biomedical research was justified as serving national purposes, rather than as a subsidy to universities.[5]

While medical school revenues from all sources were increasing throughout the 1950s, federally supported research grew more quickly than other sources and soon became the largest single source of revenue. Between 1947 and 1959, when medical school expenditures grew at about 14 percent per year, sponsored research funds grew at about 20 percent per year.[6] Federal research grants and contracts (exclusive of overhead) accounted for 19 percent of medical school revenues in 1956 to 1957, 23 percent in 1958 to 1959, and 25 percent in 1959 to 1960.[7] Sponsored research funds made up a growing proportion of medical school revenues into the 1960s. Sponsored research revenues accounted for more than 50 percent of the total increase in medical school revenues between 1947 and 1967, and federally sponsored research funding accounted for almost 85 percent of that growth.[8]

In the mid–1960s, congressional enthusiasm for the support of biomedical research began to wane. This development was due in part to the perceived failure of basic research to yield significant results and in part to growing dissatisfaction with inefficiencies in NIH's administration of biomedical research grant programs. In addition, the growing perception of a physician shortage made it necessary for Congress to divert some of the federal investment in the nation's health into the production of more physicians. As a result, the rate of increase in federal funding for biomedical research began to slow in 1964 to 1965, although it maintained a constant proportion of the gross national product into the 1980s and has often grown at a significantly faster rate than the rate of inflation.[9] Federally sponsored research peaked at about 36 percent of medical school revenues in 1963 to 1964, and this proportion declined steadily thereafter (see Table 8.1). In the early 1980s a combination of recession, the federal budget deficit, and competing federal priorities caused renewed efforts to slow the rate of increase in federal biomedical research funding. By 1984 to 1985, federally sponsored research funds represented only 14.5 percent of medical school revenues.

IMPLICATIONS OF FEDERAL BIOMEDICAL RESEARCH FUNDING

Because it subsidized the medical education enterprise only indirectly, biomedical research funding allowed the federal government to foster the growth of medical schools without directly trespassing on the profession's autonomy—that is, the medical profession's right to determine the nature of professional education and to control its growth and its quality. Nonetheless, most observers agree that during the 1950s and 1960s the character of American medical education was fundamentally altered by

Table 8.1
Major Sources of Medical School Revenue as a Proportion of Total Revenue, 1958–1988

	Federally–Funded Research (%)	Federally–Funded Training Programs (%)	Faculty Practice Plans (%)
1963–64	36.3	11.6	2.7
1966–67	34.1	12.5	3.0
1969–70	24.6	11.0	5.8
1972–73	22.4	11.2	7.3
1975–76	19.6	8.7	11.9
1978–79	18.0	4.4	11.3
1981–82	16.1	3.2	14.5
1984–85	14.5	1.9	16.6
1987–88	14.7	1.5	18.7

Source: "U.S. Medical School Finances"; *JAMA* 231 (1975): 31; 238 (1977): 2778, 262 (1989): 1023 1024.

the substantial infusion of federally sponsored research grants and their associated payments for the indirect costs of conducting research activities. Many medical schools for the first time became dependent on federal support for their educational programs, albeit indirectly through biomedical research grants. Many new full-time members were added to medical school faculties. Moreover, whereas clinically-oriented faculty members had previously been predominant, increasing numbers of faculty member now devoted greater proportions of their time to research.[10] Indirect costs associated with research grants were used to increase the number of staff, to support greater numbers of graduate students, as well as to expand medical school facilities and otherwise underwrite the costs of medical education programs. In addition, there was a notable shift in the faculty reward system; promotion and tenure criteria increasingly emphasized research productivity.[11] Stevens notes that "by 1960, the medical school was in large part a federally dominated research institution whose purpose was only partially to educate student physicians."[12]

The new dependence of many medical schools on federal biomedical research support was not without its hazards. First, the research mission threatened to overshadow the educational mission of the medical schools; it became increasingly difficult to get research-oriented faculty to participate actively in the clinical education of students. Second, many faculty members placed a higher value on research than on patient care and these values were, in turn, transmitted to students. Third, educational programs of medical schools became increasingly vulnerable to the unpredictable and unstable outcomes of federal policy and budget decision-making related to biomedical research programs. Although federal policies of the 1950s and early 1960s had not yet directly intervened in the process of medical education, by the end of this period the resources available for medical education were increasingly at the mercy of federal decision-making. However, as demonstrated in the sections that follow, growth in federal biomedical research revenues slowed as new medical school revenue appeared from other, mostly federal, sources. These included both direct federal support for the costs of training and indirect subsidy of medical education through income generated by medical care provided, mostly to Medicare and Medicaid patients, by clinical faculty members.

TRENDS IN DIRECT FEDERAL SUPPORT FOR MEDICAL EDUCATION AND MEDICAL STUDENTS

Despite growing public perceptions of a shortage of physicians, organized medicine opposed and succeeded in delaying direct federal support for medical education throughout the 1950s. The medical profession maintained its insistence that a shortage did not exist. Moreover, the profession argued that too-rapid expansion of medical schools would lower the quality of medical education.[13]

Throughout this period, a shortage of health manpower was repeatedly documented and the role of the federal government in redressing this problem was debated. Evidence from the Bayne-Jones Report in 1958, the Bane Report in 1959, and the Jones Report in 1960 persuasively documented the need for more physicians. In addition, by 1960 it became increasingly difficult to ignore the financial problems of many medical schools and the fact that many prospective medical students could not afford the rising costs of a medical education. Private and state resources were not going to be sufficient to meet these needs. By the early 1960s, the profession's efforts to maintain control over the supply of physicians and to avert federal interference in medical education began to give way to a growing sense that the federal government had a vital responsibility for assuring production of physicians at a level adequate to meet the nation's needs.[14]

The first federal provisions expressly for the purposes of medical education were included in the Health Professions Educational Assistance Act of 1963. This legislation authorized federal matching grants for constructing new and expanded medical school facilities and established a loan program for health professions students. The legislation was amended repeatedly in subsequent years, incorporating additions to the program and expanding appropriations.[15] Among the notable additions were a scholarship program for students with extreme financial need, loan-forgiveness programs for students willing to enter practice in manpower shortage areas, and a program of educational improvement grants which subsidized the operating costs of medical schools and their special programs, including activities such as curriculum development. Also notable was the institution in 1971 of capitation grants to medical schools, with payments linked to specific enrollment increases.

Various forms of federal support for medical schools and for medical students continued throughout the 1970s. By the mid–1970s the perception of a health manpower shortage was gradually replaced by concerns about an oversupply of physicians, particularly specialists, and a continuing shortage of primary care physicians. As a result, federal health manpower programs were targeted in an attempt to affect both institutional decisions (related to curriculum development) and individual student decisions (related to specialty choice). These changes were designed to meet increasingly specific national manpower objectives, such as an increase in primary care providers.

The 1976 Health Professions Educational Assistance Act extended the major federal health manpower programs until 1980. However capitation support began to be reduced in the late 1970s. With reports of an impending physician surplus, and the existence of a recession and a growing federal budget deficit, it became increasingly difficult for Congress to justify direct subsidy of medical schools. By reducing capitation support, Congress sent a message to American medical schools that they should find alternatives to direct federal subsidy of medical education. Federal capitation payments to medical schools were eliminated after 1980 and various other forms of institutional support for medical education were reduced. In addition, although federal biomedical research support increased annually during the early 1980s, the increases no longer kept pace with inflation.[16]

Various student assistance programs continued, but both the amount and the nature of federal assistance to medical students became more restricted in the 1980s.[17] These changes in the financial aid available to students have presented particular difficulties for low-income, minority, and other disadvantaged groups. Minority students, for example, are increasingly likely to graduate from college with debt. This, with the expectation of the high cost of a medical education, is thought to be discouraging medical school applications from minority students. Presently, serious concerns are being raised about future access to a medical education for disadvantaged students.[18]

During the 1980s national trends emphasized reducing federal intervention and financial commitments in most public policy areas. A similar philosophical shift was also taking place in health policy, which was moving away from government regulation and toward allowing price competition to resolve such issues as manpower maldistribution and health care price inflation. A 1981 statement by Dr. Robert Graham, acting administrator of the Department of Health and Human Services, reflects these shifts and suggests that, at least from the standpoint of the Reagan Administration, future federal intervention in medical education was not needed:

I believe that the Administration's position can be interpreted as follows: (1) The general supply of health professionals is adequate or the capacity of the U.S. health professions schools to produce the needed supply is perceived to be adequate, (2) there will be a minimum federal role for investment in terms of health professions education whether we are talking about direct project grants, institutional assistance, student aid or other support, and (3) competition will sort out the major issues of distribution, specialty choice, and workforce mix.[19]

Federal health manpower programs had created various financial incentives for medical schools to meet federal health manpower objectives. These objectives included increasing the number of American medical schools, expanding medical school enrollments, making a medical education more accessible to low-income and minority students, and increasing the numbers of primary care physicians in training.[20] Relative to other sources of revenue, the direct federal contribution to medical education was never very great. While federally-funded training programs doubled as a proportion of all medical school revenues between 1958–1959 and 1966–1967, they never reached more than 12.5 percent of revenues and they declined as a proportion of total medical schools revenues in each year since 1973 (Table 8.1).

Moreover, throughout the 1960s and 1970s, when federal health manpower programs were at their peak, direct federal support for undergraduate medical education remained a very small proportion of all federal obligations to medical schools. A 1974 report by the Committee on the Financing of Medical Education of the AAMC indicated that in 1973 only 16 percent of just over $1 billion dollars in federal obligations to medical schools supported undergraduate medical education. Eighty-four percent of the $163 million dollars allocated to undergraduate medical education in that year went toward direct institutional support (capitation grants and special project grants) and the remaining 16 percent went toward student assistance (scholarships and loans). Although support for biomedical research began to slow in the late 1960s, the overwhelming majority of federal obligations to medical schools in 1973 underwrote costs associated with the conduct of biomedical research and this pattern continued into the 1980s.[21]

IMPLICATIONS OF DIRECT FEDERAL SUPPORT FOR MEDICAL EDUCATION

Although federal health manpower programs were never a major source of medical school revenue, and although they were dwarfed in their impact by the much larger stream of biomedical research funds flowing into American medical schools, the federal health manpower programs of the 1960s and 1970s were influential in reshaping undergraduate medical education in several significant ways. These programs increased the number of medical schools, enlarged medical school enrollments, and expanded access to medical education for low-income and minority students. In addition, they fostered curriculum and faculty development in general, and the development of primary care training programs in particular, as well as attempting to bring about a more appropriate specialty mix among American physicians. Between 1963 and 1980 medical education program development received considerable attention, and the imbalance between the overdeveloped research mission and the underdeveloped educational mission of medical schools was somewhat redressed.

Withdrawal of direct federal support for health manpower programs, while the costs of medical education continued to rise, once again brought to the forefront the question how medical schools might best finance undergraduate medical education. This time, a partial answer consisted of increasingly subsidizing medical education from the growing clinical activities of faculty. In addition, many medical schools also found it necessary to raise tuition and fees. Along with declining federal assistance for medical students, this eroded many earlier gains in equity of access to a medical education.

TRENDS IN FACULTY PRACTICE PLANS

Prior to 1965, the indigent comprised most of the patient population used by medical schools for teaching and research. Medical students and residents, under the supervision of faculty members, provided care to the indigent as part of their training. This care was primarily rendered on a charity basis and subsidized by the medical school's endowment, by university funds, or by shifting the costs to paying patients. The care of the indigent was not lucrative, but it was viewed as a necessary part of medical school teaching and research. Few incentives existed for faculty to provide patient care beyond the level needed for these purposes.

The enactment of Medicare and Medicaid in 1965 converted the poor and the elderly from subsidized to paying patients, with reimbursement from the federal or state government. This development gave clinical departments in many medical schools new income, generated through the clinical activities of faculty, to offset departmental expenses. New academic group practices were created, called "faculty practice plans." These entities generated and distributed patient care revenues under policies and procedures administered by a dean, a department head, or a chief of clinical service. A 1977 study of faculty practice plans found that 70 percent of these plans were implemented after 1960. Between 1960 and 1985 the number of faculty practice plans increased from 6 to 118. As of the mid–1980s, 118 (93 percent) of the 127 U.S. medical schools had faculty practice plans.[22]

Faculty practice plans contributed a relatively small proportion of medical school revenues until the late 1960s. However, between 1972–1973 and 1987–1988 the proportion of medical school revenues derived from faculty practice plans more than doubled (Table 8.1). Throughout this period, revenue from faculty practice plans grew from year to year, sometimes increasing by as much as 35 to 50 percent in a given year (Table 8.2).

While Medicare and Medicaid paved the way for the development of faculty practice plans, other factors also contributed to their dramatic emergence as a source of medical school revenue throughout the 1970s and 1980s. Most important were the declining availability of federal biomedical research funds and, subsequently, the dwindling of direct federal support for medical education. These developments made it necessary for medical schools to find new sources of support for the faculty hired and the programs initiated with the federal funding of the 1960s and early 1970s. Increasing income from faculty clinical activities throughout the 1970s and 1980s has enabled medical schools to soften the impact of declining federal support for biomedical research and for medical education.

CURRENT STATUS OF FACULTY PRACTICE PLANS

A study by MacLeod and Schwarz documented the great variability of faculty practice plans. In some schools the faculty practice plan encompassed only one department and as few as six faculty members; in other schools as many as twenty-five departments and 950 faculty members participated. Most often some eleven to fifteen departments participated. Basic science departments (except pathology) were rarely involved; medicine, obstetrics and gynecology, pediatrics, psychiatry, ra-

Table 8.2
Percentage Increases in Medical School Revenues from Professional Fee Income

Years	Percentage Increase
1961–62 to 1962–63	7.6
1964–65 to 1965–66	15.4
1967–68 to 1968–69	35.4
1970–71 to 1971–72	19.1
1973–74 to 1974–75	50.7
1976–77 to 1977–78	9.3
1979–80 to 1980–81	24.5
1982–83 to 1983–84	12.7
1985–86 to 1986–87	15.0
1986–87 to 1987–88	19.0

Source: "U.S. Medical School Finances"; *JAMA* 190 (1964): 616; 231 (1975): 31; 238 (1977): 2778; 258 (1987): 1026; 262 (1989): 1023.

diology, and surgery were almost always included. About 70 percent of faculty practice plans were tax-exempt, not-for-profit corporations; the remaining 30 percent were either for-profit corporations, or had some mixture of not-for-profit and for-profit status.

The governance structures of faculty practice plans varied widely as did the structures used to administer the plan. Plans also varied in the power over policies and administration accorded to the medical school dean and in the relative power accorded to participating departments. These differences were expressed in the specific arrangements for the distribution of clinical revenues. However, while plans differed in their specifics, in most cases the general mechanism for distributing plan income was the same: first, monies were set aside to cover the costs of administering the plan; second, a proportion (varying from plan to plan) was allocated to the dean for discretionary use in supporting medical school programs; finally, remaining revenue was allocated among clinical faculty according to a predetermined formula generally designed to reward clinical productivity.[23]

IMPACT OF FACULTY PRACTICE PLANS ON MEDICAL EDUCATION

The emergence of faculty practice plans set into motion interlocking developments which once again transformed the shape of medical schools, medical faculties, and medical education. First, faculty practice plan income was used to hire more full-time clinical faculty members to provide patient care, supplanting the role of the traditional part-time faculty members in many schools.[24] In contrast with the earlier part-time clinical faculty who voluntarily contributed their time to the supervision of students and to the care of the indigent, many of the newly hired clinical faculty had little or no private practice experience. As a result, students were now increasingly under the supervision of clinical faculty members whose practice experience was limited to the teaching hospital. Less of the unique wisdom of the generalist private practitioner was being included in clinical training.[25]

Second, since Medicare and Medicaid now reimbursed faculty for their hands-on care of the elderly and the poor, these activities became more lucrative. Thus, many patient care activities formerly delegated to medical students and residents were gradually usurped by clinical faculty. These developments altered students' clinical experiences: on the one hand, students now had more contact with and supervision from experienced clinicians; on the other hand, some opportunities for students to develop autonomy and independent decision-making were lost.[26]

Third, since significant income could be derived from clinical practice, medical schools had to make greater efforts to offer clinical faculty members salaries competitive with those available in private practice. As a result of growing numbers of clinical faculty, rising faculty salaries, and the administrative costs of billing and collections for the faculty practice plan, expenses of clinical departments grew, making it necessary for clinical faculty to generate ever increasing amounts of clinical revenue. Thus, clinical care came to dominate the concerns of many clinical faculty, all but overshadowing their teaching activities. During the biomedical research heyday of the 1950s and 1960s, it had sometimes been difficult to lure research-oriented faculty away from their laboratories to teach clinical skills to medical students. In the late 1960s and early 1970s, as faculty practice plans began to grow, relatively more faculty became actively involved in patient care. As pressure to generate patient care revenues also grew, these clinical faculty, like their research-oriented counterparts, also found they had little time for teaching.[27]

Finally, although faculty practice plans evolved slowly and their characteristics varied considerably, in most schools departmental growth was now tied closely to the department's service capability. Although plan revenues were to some extent used to cross-subsidize medical school departments, most revenue was returned to the generating department for its own use. As a result, relatively little of the revenue was allocated to the basic science departments, to clinical departments in the primary care specialties, and to departments whose clinicians specialized in cognitive rather than procedural medical interventions. Departments of medicine and surgery grew; within them, substantial sums were allocated to support the facilities and the faculties of the highest-revenue-generating subspecialties. Most of the unequal growth of medical school departments occurring as a result of the rise of faculty practice plans was driven by the vagaries of a third-party reimbursement system which paid relatively more for high levels of medical technology, for medical procedures, and for subspecialty services.[28] Little of the uneven growth of medical school departments was related to any planned attempt to fulfill the educational needs of physicians in training.

IMPLICATIONS OF FACULTY PRACTICE PLANS: PRESENT AND FUTURE

As noted earlier, faculty practice plans grew rapidly in an ad hoc and largely unplanned way. Medical schools created these plans as a response to the changing fiscal environment, but little thought was given to the implications of faculty practice plans for the medical schools themselves or for the enterprise of medical education. Recently, however, the continuing growth of faculty practice plans has begun to raise many challenging and controversial issues. These issues are currently being debated and their resolution will have important implications for the future shape of medical education. In general, this debate assumes that faculty practice plans are here to stay. It is viewed as unlikely that the future will bring a substantial resurgence of federal support for biomedical research and for medical education. There are few alternatives seen to the revenue generated by faculty from clinical practice. As a result, most of the current debate centers on how faculty practice plans can best be constituted to support medical schools and medical education, at present and in the future.

Many of the issues being debated relate to plan administration. One important question is the degree to which administrative decision-making should be either centralized with the dean or decentralized to the departmental level. Presumably, the dean is in the best position to plan and make decisions with the best interests of the whole medical school in mind. However, since most faculty practice plans were originally organized at the departmental level, and since many medical schools deans possess little authority over the departments, it can be difficult to establish centralized control of the faculty practice plan.

As a result of the decentralized decision-making which characterizes most plans, little explicit control is exercised over how much time clinical faculty spend in direct patient care.[29] With strong departmental expectations for clinical faculty to generate revenue, accompanied by the financial incentives associated with doing so, both teaching and scholarly activities tend to be minimized. This has led some observers to question whether new arrangements may be needed to ensure that the clinical teaching function of faculty is somehow preserved. Some argue that the faculty reward system needs to be adjusted so that faculty are duly rewarded for excellence in clinical teaching.[30] Others argue that productive clinical faculty should be exempted from teaching and that a separate category of "clinician/teacher" is needed.[31] Still others argue for the possible return of the part-time clinical faculty member with a commitment to education and a willingness to teach.[32]

The emergence of larger clinical faculties with substantial patient care responsibilities has also called into question the adequacy of existing criteria for medical school faculty appointment, promotion, and tenure. Many observers recognize that the existing reward system, which values research and scholarship most highly, is inadequate to accommodate the increasing diversity of talent represented among medical school faculty members.[33] As long as a uni-dimensional, research-oriented reward system endures, young clinical faculty face only dim prospects for advancement. Similarly, as long as clinical teaching remains unrewarded, it is unlikely to receive the serious attention of clinical faculty. The need for more adequate academic rewards for clinical excellence is widely appreciated. However, inertia, as well as powerful conservative faculty members who have tended to hold research in the highest regard, has forestalled the needed changes in the reward system of many medical schools.

Most fundamental, controversial, and challenging are questions related to the distribution of plan income. This affects every aspect of medical school operations, determining how much clinical revenue will be used to support educational programs, which departments will grow and flourish, which faculty members will grow wealthier, and which departments may have to eliminate faculty positions and curtail such faculty privileges as financial support for travel to professional meetings. Historically, decisions about the allocation of plan income have resulted in the growth of medical school clinical departments, the withering of many basic science departments, and the relative wealth of the medical and surgical subspecialty faculties in comparison to their primary care counterparts.[34] Such allocation decisions also shape the clinical services of teaching hospitals and academic medical centers as pressures mount to drop services producing too little revenue (such as home care, family planning, burn units, rehabilitation units, and care of the uninsured) and to expand those services with the greatest revenue-generating potential (such as open-heart surgery units, intensive care units, pathology and cardiac catheterization laboratories).[35]

The relative decision-making power of the dean and the departments in allocating plan income is among the questions most hotly debated. Some observers call for a greater degree of centralized decision-making, arguing that this is the best way to ensure an equitable distribution tied closely to the overall goals of the institution. Others suggest that such centralization violates faculty autonomy and destroys incentives for clinical productivity. Similarly controversial are questions of the degree to which departments should subsidize one another and the degree to which clinical revenue should be taxed to support educational programs, student scholarships, non-lucrative services, and other overarching educational and service objectives of the institution. A 1985 survey of medical schools' leaders conducted by the AAMC found that these were considered to be among the most important issues currently facing faculty practice plans.[36]

As faculty practice plans have grown, medical school departments have become increasingly businesslike. Management challenges abound. Successful administration of faculty practice plans requires careful attention to matters such as cash flow, billing, and collections. Faculty are increasing called upon to develop new marketing strategies and referral networks which will help to increase revenues. During the mid–1980s, with keener competition in the health care sector, faculty practice plans increasingly contemplated developing (or affiliating with) health maintenance organizations (HMOs), independent practice associations (IPAs), and preferred provider organizations (PPOs).[37]

Stemmler has noted that many medical schools do not presently have the managerial strength needed to compete effectively in today's competitive health care environment; the power and decision-making in faculty practice plans tend to be too decentralized and the cost containment incentives governing clinical practice tend to be too weak.[38] Some observers note that if they are to thrive, faculty practice plans will need to "be reorganized into 'true group practices,' with coordinated management of patients, internal referral systems, and mechanisms to negotiate as a group with HMOs and PPOs for brokered care."[39]

In addition to the demands of an increasingly competitive health care environment, faculty practice plans also now face the vagaries of the changing third-party reimbursement system. One such change was Medicare's implementation in the early 1980s of a prospective hospital payment system based on diagnosis-related groups (DRGs). Many state Medicaid programs also now use a DRG system for hospital reimbursement. Since most faculty practice plans derive their income from reimbursement for physician's services, the impact of DRGs on faculty practice plans was not as severe as was their impact on teaching hospitals.

However, Stemmler argues that DRGs have to some extent placed faculty practice plans at odds with the teaching hospitals. For example, faculty practice plans now have increasing incentives to set up and operate freestanding diagnostic facilities while "allowing the hospital's diagnostic unit to become relatively underutilized."[40] Such divergence in the interests of faculty practice plans and the teaching hospitals with which they are affiliated threatens to unravel the fabric of academic medical centers.

While DRGs primarily affected hospitals, other Medicare and Medicaid policy changes have altered the ways in which physicians' services are reimbursed. Physician reimbursement has become increasingly restrictive, caps have been placed on the Medicare payment levels for particular services, and the search is presently under way for a new system to replace Medicare's usual, customary, and reasonable (UCR) method of reimbursing physicians. One proposed system would institute physician reimbursement based on a resource based relative value scale (RBRVS) which would weigh reimbursement levels according to the time and effort expended in providing the service. Such a system would dramatically alter the amount paid for different physician services: relatively more money would be paid for the so-called "cognitive services" (such as office visits) and relatively less would be paid for the so-called "procedural services" (such as cataract surgery). Such a change in the third-party reimbursement system would have untold effects on the total revenue generated by faculty practice plans, as well as on the revenue-generating potential of particular clinical departments.

The potential dangers of relying on clinical income to subsidize medical education were forecast by Fein and Weber. In 1971, they observed:

Some medical schools are expressing concern that they may once again be embarking on a dangerous route: a route where their educational mission is supported out of funds generated by another activity (this time service rather than research). Though this type of support may prove helpful, the danger is that once again national priorities may change and the school's service-derived funds may be cut.[41]

The kinds of cutbacks Fein and Weber envisioned have indeed taken place: in the 1980s both Medicare and Medicaid reduced program entitlements and instituted various cost containment strategies which have threatened to limit the revenue generating potential of medical school clinical faculty. This threat is likely to continue and faculty practice plans will need to plan carefully to protect educational programs from the uncertainties of third-party reimbursement policy.

The trend toward increasing reliance of medical schools on faculty practice plan income raises fundamental philosophical questions. For example, once again, as during the earlier era when biomedical research funds were being used to support medical education, serious concerns are being raised about the fate of the medical school's educational mission. With so many programmatic and service decisions being driven by the need to generate clinical income, relatively little weight seems to be given to decisions which would foster the development of excellence in medical education. Some authors decry the shift away from the research mission and toward the service mission as a seeming return to the pre-Flexnerian era of clinically-oriented, proprietary medical schools.[42] Others, like Cluff, observe that the problem created by increased faculty responsibility for patient care "comes not from the use of practice income, which forms the base for faculty practice plans to meet the financial needs of medical schools, but from the incentive to divert efforts away from education to increase revenues."[43] Resolution of this problem will require that the medical schools counterbalance concerns for revenue with concerns for overarching educational objectives.

A similar philosophical question is raised as medical school faculty and their teaching hospitals allow themselves to be diverted from the care of the indigent and the provision of "socially relevant" services, which may produce little revenue but are, nonetheless, needed by the surrounding community. Academic medical centers and their component faculties have a long history of providing medical care to the indigent and otherwise meeting the health care needs of the underserved. Sustaining this commitment will require that medical schools counterbalance growing concerns for revenue with concerns for the attainment of social objectives.

CONCLUSION

Throughout recent decades, the undergraduate medical education enterprise has generally been subsidized with revenues obtained by medical schools for other purposes, such as biomedical research and, more recently, patient care. The major exception to this history of cross-subsidization was of a brief period of direct federal support for medical schools during the 1960s and 1970s, a period in which the instruments of public policy were used to help expand the number of U.S. medical schools and to increase the nation's supply of health manpower. Recently, however, federal policy has retreated from the task of subsidizing medical schools: federal biomedical research programs have been reduced, direct support in the form of capitation grants has been eliminated, some student loan and scholarship programs have been eliminated, and the terms of other programs of financial support for medical students have become more financially onerous.

The major adaptation medical schools have made to declining federal support has been to increase revenue from patient care and to use some of the revenue generated from clinical activities to support educational programs. This adaptative strategy has enabled medical schools to shift away from their earlier institutional emphases on research and scholarship. The organizational goals of many medical schools have shifted dramatically toward service and a certain amount of confusion has been created in the process. As described earlier, medical schools now struggle with such fundamental decisions as how best to reward both scholarship and clinical excellence, how to compete most effectively in a competitive medical marketplace, and how to organize and manage faculty practice plans to maximize clinical revenue and support the diverse programs of the medical school. At this point in their history, the development of adequate clinical revenue by many medical schools continues to be a matter of survival. It is unlikely that large amounts of federal support for medical schools will be available in the future and, as a result, medical schools continue to face the twin challenges of developing well-managed faculty practice plans and developing other alternatives to federal financial support.

The recent history of medical school financing suggests that undergraduate medical education has often been the step-child of the medical school, receiving somewhat lower priority than either research or, more recently, patient care. As we have been seen, one current implication of cross-subsidization is that medical school faculty and curricula are to some extent being shaped more by the demands of patient care than by the needs of medical education per se. The future of undergraduate medical education will depend largely on reconciling these sometimes conflicting demands. Embedded in decisions about faculty recruitment, faculty reward systems, and the allocation of clinical revenues are a medical school's value judgments about the importance of educational programs relative to other activities, about the importance of providing support for student scholarships and loans to facilitate continued access of disadvantaged students to a medical education, and about the institution's commitment to maintaining non-lucrative medical services of important social value to the surrounding community. Thus, perhaps the single most challenge now facing many medical schools is that of harnessing the resources of faculty practice plans to serve the best interests of medical education, medical schools, and the surrounding community.

9

Trends in the Use of Outpatient Settings for Medical Education

Barbara Barzansky and Janet D. Perloff

There has been clinical teaching in outpatient settings throughout the century, but the curricular placement and extent of outpatient clinical experiences have varied over time. From being the major site for student contact with patients before 1920, the outpatient setting fell into relative disfavor during the 1960s and 1970s. There currently is a movement to expand outpatient teaching, but the degree to which this change has been implemented is variable among clinical disciplines and medical schools.

"Outpatient care" and "ambulatory care" (the more current term) often are used synonomously. However, outpatient care historically has been defined more broadly. For example, it includes non-ambulatory patients in their homes. A wide variety of sites of care have been used for outpatient teaching, such as the clinics (dispensaries) of medical school teaching hospitals, the offices of community practitioners, the homes of patients, and the facilities of prepaid health plans (such as HMOs). These various sites have some characteristics in common, but also some differences that are important for educational purposes.

OUTPATIENT TEACHING IN HOSPITAL CLINICS, 1900 TO 1950

At the time of the "Flexner Report," only a few medical schools had instituted a clerkship that included active student participation in the care of patients. More often, students received clinical instruction by visiting the wards of hospitals for demonstrations. In the better schools, this activity occurred in small groups.[1] To supplement such didactic clinical teaching, medical schools used outpatient clinics (dispensaries) to introduce students to the diagnosis of common clinical problems. In the early part of the century, outpatient work was predominantly located in the third year of the curriculum and inpatient teaching in the fourth year. For example, at the turn of the century at Johns Hopkins School of Medicine, third-year courses in the Department of Medicine included an observation clinic, which met three times a week for one hour in a classroom associated with the outpatient department. The entire class attended, and students took turns examining patients. Students were required to follow up their patients, visiting them in the hospital or in their homes. In addition, physical diagnosis and history-taking mainly were taught using clinic patients. Students also participated in the General Medical Clinic, in which the common diseases of the day (such as typhoid and pneumonia) were demonstrated and discussed. William Osler, in describing the Johns Hopkins program, advocated the use of the ambulatory clinic because "the student sees close at hand the unwashed maladies, not the distant prepared and altered picture of the amphitheater."[2]

A special committee of the AMA's CME, charged with developing a plan for the reorganization of clinical teaching, described their view of the optimal use of outpatient clinics in a 1915 report. The ten-member committee of prominent physicians proposed that clinical studies should begin with practical exercises in the study of physical signs and their relation to symptoms and pathologic processes (an exercise similar to the John Hopkins observation clinic). This exercise should occur in the second year using normal subjects or clinic patients. Practical work in the clinic and at the bedside should occupy the third year, accompanied by didactic teaching and formal (demonstration and discussion) clinics and lectures. Clerkships should be placed in the fourth year. The outpatient clinic was especially recommended for teaching internal medicine and the medical specialties, ophthalmology, otology, and rhinolaryngology. Fourth-year students should have opportunities to care for obstetrical patients, both in the hospital and in the patient's home.[3]

A similar pattern of outpatient instruction was being implemented by leading clinical educators. George Dock of Washington University in St. Louis wrote that he initially had reservations about teaching basic clinical skills in the clinic, because he "feared the superficial methods fostered by dispensary needs." He was, however, convinced by the arguments of Osler, with whom he had "had heated arguments on the subject." Later Dock came to praise the level of skills that students could acquire in the clinics. Dock took care to organize the clinic space to facilitate teaching, provided adequate student supervision, and arranged patient attendance to minimize waiting and allow sufficient time for examinations.[4]

The "superficial methods of the dispensary" were a problem in many institutions using clinics for student teaching. Some commentators felt that the treatment of patients in outpatient departments was inferior to the care provided in the wards. This was because the patient volume was high and the time available for each patient was short, so that methods of examination were superficial and the treatments prescribed were routine. William Rothstein has noted

ambulatory patients had long waits, regardless of their jobs or family responsibilities, and those with little understanding of English were seldom given language assistance. The overburdened and unpaid physician tended to ask a few questions, prescribe a drug or two, and dismiss the patient.[5]

Another source of problems was that there was essentially a "two-class" system for clinical faculty members. The outpatient physicians usually were part-time junior faculty members and they often had little contact with the members of their departments who provided inpatient care. In addition, clinic facilities often were unsatisfactory and medical records were sketchy.[6]

These negative conditions made for less than optimal teaching experiences for both students and faculty members. As time progressed, outpatient teaching was moved from the second and third years of the curriculum into the fourth year, the argument being that students could learn basic skills better in the more controlled environment of the wards.[7] The 1932 *Final Report* of the Commission on Medical Education, while reiterating some of the problems with outpatient teaching that already have been described, stressed the importance of the setting in preparing students for their future practice. The report recommended that teaching be done by senior members of the faculty and staff, and that opportunities be provided for follow-up of clinic patients in the wards or at home.[8]

By the mid- to late-1930s, about half of medical schools still assigned third-year medical students to outpatient clinics in the various specialties, and the remainder had moved outpatient teaching to the fourth year. The quality of outpatient instruction was variable, with some schools having inadequate facilities and providing insufficient supervision of students. An inadequate number of patients for teaching was a problem in some surgical clinics. For obstetrics, more than two-thirds of schools had home delivery services. This practice was being threatened, however, by the increased tendency for women to have their babies in the hospital.[9]

The curricular shift of the inpatient clinical clerkship to the third year was about complete by 1950. The fourth year was devoted to outpatient teaching and instruction in the specialties. Students often rotated through as many as ten to fifteen general and special clinics, spending only a few weeks in each.

At mid-century, there was dissatisfaction arising from the fragmented organization of outpatient departments. There could be twenty-five to thirty individual clinics in a large outpatient department, making continuity of care and communication difficult if not impossible. Many clinic physicians served on a volunteer basis, caring for a large number of patients and simultaneously trying to teach students. In addition, the status and perceived utility of the clinics remained low. The outpatient department was considered by administrators and senior clinical faculty members to be secondary to the inpatient service. In their opinions, the main use of the clinics was for selecting interesting patients for ward teaching.[10]

In summary, during the first half of the twentieth century outpatient teaching moved from the second and third years of the curriculum to the fourth year. The focus of outpatient teaching shifted from the acquisition of clinical skills to more specialty-oriented experiences. Many problems were identified with the use of medical school outpatient clinics for teaching. In response, other models of outpatient teaching began to be introduced to supplement instruction in the clinics.

THE PRECEPTORSHIP

Preceptorships involve a one-to-one educational experience, with students spending time with practicing physicians in their offices and participating in their regular patient care activities. An extended preceptorship (apprenticeship) was the major format of medical education until about the middle of the nineteenth century. With the increase in the number of medical schools, the apprenticeship model of medical education disappeared, only to re-emerge later in a shortened and modified form. This initial reappearance occurred in the 1920s, when a few medical schools such as the University of Wisconsin instituted short-duration preceptorships.

The number of schools with preceptorships gradually increased during the late 1940s and early 1950s. There were nine programs in 1948 and twenty-four in 1954. In only about one-half of these schools was the preceptorship required. There also was some turnover of programs. In 1954, only four programs had been in existence for more than five years.[11]

Preceptorships were structured so that students spent from two weeks to three months (average six weeks in 1952) at the office of a physician usually in a small town at a distance from the medical school. Preceptorships most commonly occurred in the summer between the third and fourth years or during the fourth year.[12] In the 1950s, physicians chosen as preceptors were usually general practitioners, and the objectives of the preceptorship often included acquainting students with general practice as a way of life.[13]

By the mid–1960s, the number of schools with preceptorships had increased (to thirty-four in 1964) but the total number of participating students had decreased. About 70 percent of medical schools with preceptorship programs were state supported. An explicit purpose of these preceptorships was to influence the distribution of health manpower by introducing students to practice in rural locations.[14]

Descriptions of individual programs from the 1950s through the 1980s reveal many similarities. A major objective of the rural preceptorship program at the University of Kansas during the 1950s was for the student to "contemplate the physician's role in society as well as his social and civic responsibilities." This program used towns of fewer than 2,500 as preceptorship sites. Students spent five and one-half weeks making house calls with their preceptors, participating in hospital rounds, and taking an active part in office routine. It also was expected that students share in the personal lives of their preceptors, and students often lived in their preceptors' homes.[15]

In the early 1970s, the Rural Physician Associate Program (RPAP) was established at the University of Minnesota Medical School in response to a legislative mandate to develop a program to replenish the supply of general physicians in rural Minnesota. The RPAP was a nine- to twelve-month elective experience for third year-students, with an average of thirty-three students participating per year. The goals of the program were to influence students to practice in rural Minnesota; to allow students to experience the work and life style of physicians and their families in rural settings; and to provide an awareness of behavioral, psychological, preventive, and environmental factors in patient care. About 98 percent of preceptors were board-certified, and the majority came from the disciplines of family medicine, internal medicine, and pediatrics.[16]

Students in the University of New Mexico School of Medicine Primary Care Curriculum in the 1980s spent sixteen weeks during the second half of the first year with a primary care physician (in family medicine, internal medicine, or pediatrics). The preceptorships were located throughout the state. The goals of the program were to provide students with: (1) a balance of clinical experiences reflecting the world of practice, (2) a "real-life" context for learning relevant social sciences, and (3) skills in working with other health professionals and community representatives. Students spent about one-half of the time in a patient care setting and the rest in independent study.[17]

In summary, these programs share the goals of introducing students to the realities of medical practice and the physician's role in the larger society. A commentator in the 1950s remarked that in very few cases was the preceptorship expected to contribute to the students' "fundamental knowledge in medicine."[18] The perception that preceptorships had no significant cognitive value gave them a negative image among those who saw medical education as synonomous with mastering biomedical knowledge. Other problems identified with the preceptorship included variability in the content and quality of medical student experiences (for example, students given too little or too much clinical responsibility), difficulty in monitoring students and preceptors, and variation in the instructional skills of preceptors.[19] To counter these problems, medical schools with well developed programs carefully selected and trained preceptors and sent faculty members or administrators to visit preceptorial sites on a regular basis.[20]

COMPREHENSIVE CARE PROGRAMS

Comprehensive medical care was defined as the organized provision of health services to families, including the full spectrum of services from prevention through rehabilitation, continuity of care for the individual, emphasis on the social and personal aspects of disease and its management, and the use of the health team concept with personal physician responsibility.[21] In the 1950s, concern with the quality of education in hospital outpatient clinics, plus a reaction to the growing emphasis on inpatient medicine and specialism, led some medical schools to develop comprehensive care programs. While most of the programs lasted less than a decade, many of the elements of comprehensive care re-emerged later in family and community medicine.[22]

About twenty medical schools introduced educational programs in clinics that included some aspects of comprehensive care, but only a few of these clinics were organized primarily to achieve the joint goals of providing comprehensive care to patients and teaching the principles of comprehensive care to students.[23] Two of these programs will be described.

The Cornell University Medical College program was initiated in 1952. It consisted of a twenty-two week clerkship in ambulatory medicine, pediatrics, public health, and psychiatry for fourth-year students. The student spent two half-days per week in the general medicine clinic for all twenty-two weeks, two half-days per week in the psychiatry clinic for eleven weeks, and two half-days per week in the pediatrics clinic for eleven weeks. Two half-days per week were spent in elective clinics and three half-days were devoted to conferences, grand rounds, and other didactic activities. An additional two half-days per week were devoted to seminars and free time that could be used for research, home visits, and preparation of a senior thesis. Each student was assigned either family care or home care patients, for long-term follow-up during the rotation.[24]

The program was organized non-departmentally, in that it was responsible to the joint administrative board of the medical center. The president of the board appointed an advisory committee, which included clinical service chiefs, the director of social service, the dean of the nursing school, the superintendent of the hospital, the chair of the outpatient department, and the professor of preventive medicine. Until 1960, the program was supported by foundation funding. After that time, various departments supported individual personnel. This change in the funding pattern, as well as negative attitudes of certain clinical faculty members, led to the reduction and then elimination of the program during a curriculum change in 1969 that made the fourth year of the curriculum elective.[25]

The University of Colorado School of Medicine, in conjunction with the Denver General Hospital, established a General Medical Clinic to provide comprehensive care in 1952. The purpose of the educational program was to ensure that students learned as much basic medical knowledge as students in traditional specialty clinics, while acquiring additional knowledge and skills in the psychological and sociological areas fundamental to comprehensive care. The General Medical Clinic was staffed by faculty members from internal medicine and pediatrics, with consultants from obstetrics-gynecology, preventive medicine, psychiatry, and surgery.

A research component was an integral part of the implementation plan. Therefore, for the first five years of the project, one-half of the fourth-year class was assigned to the General Medical Clinic and the other half was assigned to the regular clinics. The "experimental" group spent five half-days per week for eighteen weeks and two half-days per week for six weeks in the General Medical Clinic. There was a family care component of the program, so that when a new General Medical Clinic patient was assigned to a student, he/she became responsible for the care of the other family members as well.

After five years, the research component was completed and all fourth-year students were assigned to the General Medical Clinic for three half-days per week. The clinic was eliminated in 1961, when the affiliation between the Denver General Hospital and the medical school was dissolved.

An evaluation at the end of the first five years showed that the traditional medical knowledge and skills of the students in the General Medical Clinic were equivalent to what students in the regular clinics possessed. However, the experimental group had only a slight increase in psychological and sociological knowledge and skills. There were logistical problems that may have contributed to this outcome. First, the patient population was not ideal. Patients had serious chronic disease and overwhelming social problems. Also many of the patients came from unstable families, compromising the family-care component of the program.[26]

In summary, these and other comprehensive medicine programs sought to overcome the fragmented experience in traditional ambulatory care clinics by providing a relatively long-term, integrated outpatient experience. Problems that led to the disappearance of these programs were organizational (including financing), attitudinal (resistance of many clinical faculty members), and logistical (difficulties finding families suitable for medical students). Student attitudes toward these programs were generally favorable.[27]

PREPAID HEALTH CARE SETTINGS (HMOs)

The health maintenance organization (HMO) provides a comprehensive set of health services in return for a fixed prospective periodic payment.[28] The increase in the number of HMOs in the early 1970s led to consideration of their usefulness as sites for outpatient education. There are certain unique features of HMOs that made this an attractive possibility, including the emphasis on comprehensive longitudinal care and on the efficient (cost-effective) use of health services. Both these elements are weak or absent in the traditional hospital outpatient clinic setting.

Although the concept of using HMOs for outpatient teaching is appealing, the actual amount of usage has been low. A 1973 survey revealed that of thirty-four operational or planned HMOs associated with academic health centers, more than 50 percent had no medical student teaching programs or had educational experiences that involved less than five percent of the class. Only five operational or planned HMOs had educational programs that would involve all students in a given medical school.[29]

This minor involvement in teaching did not increase over time. Data from a 1982 survey showed that twenty-six medical schools (21 percent of respondents) had a formal arrangement with one or more HMOs for medical student training. In fourteen of the twenty-six schools, some third-year students took required clerkships or seminars, and in eighteen of the schools some-fourth year students took elective clerkships at the HMO. In most cases, only a small percentage of students were involved in clinical experiences at the HMOs.[30]

With the increasing number of HMOs, it is logical to ask why the level of involvement in teaching has been relatively low. One major factor has to do with costs. Medical students do not "pay their way" by providing extensive clinical service, and the instructional time that they require competes with patient care. In a 1986 study, the cost of medical student education was calculated to be about $17,000 per full-time-equivalent student per year. HMO administrators are reluctant to finance these increased costs from members payments. However, this problem has been overcome in some cases by medical schools making payments to the HMO to defray the educational costs. Subjective benefits to the HMO from a teaching program were identified to be increased quality of patient care, increased physician learning, and increased patient satisfaction.[31]

THE CURRENT STATUS OF OUTPATIENT TEACHING

In the 1970s, with the conversion of most schools to an elective fourth year, the amount of outpatient teaching in the required curriculum decreased. Ambulatory care experiences were mainly found in discrete primary care clerkships and included as part of regular required third-year clerkships.

In 1973, seventy-two medical schools (69 percent of those responding to a survey) had a required ambulatory care experience and thirty-three (31 percent of respondents) did not. In ten schools, the experience was less than one month in length and in thirty-one schools it was longer than two months.[32] In a 1976 follow-up survey, 82 percent of responding schools had a required ambulatory experience. Between 1973 and 1976, the percentage of medical schools where the majority of medical students had ambulatory care experiences in a non-hospital setting (community clinics, satellite medical centers, physicians' offices) increased. In 1973, 75 percent or more of students had such "off-campus" experiences in slightly more than one-third of medical schools; in 1976, 75 percent or more of students had such experiences in more than one-half of medical schools.[33] In 1989, 119 medical schools (94 percent of the total) offered an ambulatory primary care clerkship for students.[34]

Also in 1989, students had ambulatory experiences within the required third-year clerkships. However, the percentage of time spent in outpatient settings varied considerably across clerkships. An average of 80 percent of time in required family medicine clerkships was spent in the outpatient setting, 37 percent of time in pediatrics clerkships, 29 percent of time in obstetrics-gynecology clerkships, 18 percent of time in psychiatry clerkships, 13 percent of time in surgery clerkships, and 9 percent of time in internal medicine clerkships. The variation among disciplines is striking. In about 70 percent of required family medicine clerkships, students spent 75 percent or more of the time in the outpatient setting; in 50 percent of internal medicine clerkships, students spent no time in the outpatient setting.[35]

UNIQUE CHARACTERISTICS OF OUTPATIENT SETTINGS

The outpatient setting always has, to some degree, been used for the clinical education of medical students. Why, then, is there currently such intense discussion about increasing ambulatory care teaching?

Commentators agree that changes in the health care delivery system have made the inpatient services of hospitals less ideal as sites for clinical teaching then they once were. The increased emphasis on cost containment by major purchasers of health care has led to shorter hospital stays and to initial diagnostic workups being performed on an outpatient basis. This has diminished the previous opportunity for students to observe the natural history of disease in their hospitalized patients and to develop their own diagnostic impressions. In addition, now hospitalized patients are critically ill, and often suffer from multiple complex problems. If the goal of third-year clerkships is to teach basic knowledge and skills, these patients may not be the most appropriate for students to work with.[36]

In addition, it is argued that students should be given the opportunity to learn in a setting that resembles the actual sites where they eventually will be providing patient care. The validity of this argument depends on demonstrating that educational experiences in ambulatory care settings are in some ways different from experiences in the hospital, and that these differences reflect the "real world" of medical practice. A number of authors have described some of these unique characteristics of ambulatory care settings.[37] First, these settings provide experience with the natural history of disease. Patients often present with initial symptoms, and the physician must determine if these represent the beginning of a serious disease process. In a long-term relationship, the physician follows the patient through the course of the disease, and if the condition is chronic, provides ongoing care.

Also, the hospital inpatient setting includes only a small subset of medical problems. Individuals with minor diseases may never enter the hospital, and those with chronic disease may be admitted only during serious episodes. The outpatient setting includes a broader spectrum of patients, from those with serious organic illness to those with manifestations of psychosocial problems.

An important emphasis of outpatient care is on prevention and social medicine. Inpatient hospital care is concerned with curing a specific episode of illness. Outpatient care, especially if it is ongoing, is involved in recognizing sources of potential danger in the patient's lifestyle and in alleviating problem behaviors. In addition, the impact of disease on the patient and the patient's family are more evident in outpatient care.

Finally, communication and interpersonal interaction skills are especially important. Outpatients are more in control of their care than hospital inpatients. They can refuse to return or to comply with physician recommendations. This makes communication and negotiation critical to good patient care.

While these differences are intuitively obvious, it is logical to ask whether students do, in fact, "learn something different" by being in the ambulatory care setting. There is some evidence to indicate that this is the case. One study comparing students in a nine-month rural preceptorship with students in traditional hospital based clerkships showed differences in the types of clinical problems seen, the numbers and kinds of clinical skills and minor procedures performed, and the level of student responsibility for primary clinical problems.[38]

While outpatient settings (for example, the office of a rural practitioner, an HMO, the ophthalmology clinic of an urban teaching hospital) share some similarities, they differ in a number of important ways. One major similarity is that patients are available for relatively short periods of time. This requires efficient patient management and the ability to prioritize. The various settings differ in presenting patient problems, potential for continuity of care, incentives for cost efficient use of resources, participation of other health professionals, and emphasis on the psychosocial (in addition to the biomedical) aspects of illness.

These differences have important implications for the education of medical students. That is, settings should be chosen to meet specific objectives. For example, if the objective is to give students experience with continuity of care, a practitioner's office or an HMO might be selected. The student also would have to spend enough time in the setting for continuity to be demonstrated. If the objective is to teach the management of chronic illness, a medical school specialty clinic (for hypertension or diabetes) or a practitioner's office might be selected. The cost-effective use of resources might best be presented in an HMO, while the importance of the patient's environment and support systems could be demonstrated through home visits. It is necessary that educational planners not consider the outpatient setting as a unitary phenomenon. The objectives to be met through outpatient teaching should first be identified, and then appropriate sites to match these objectives should be chosen.

OVERCOMING BARRIERS TO THE USE OF AMBULATORY CARE SETTINGS FOR TEACHING

The factors that have affected the use of ambulatory care settings in the past have included: (1) the low status of the settings, and the "second class" position of physician-teachers in the clinics; (2) the difficulty of managing teaching in a busy setting with patients available for only a short time; and (3) the costs (in terms of time lost) associated with teaching. These same factors are being described as barriers today.[39]

What can overcome these disincentives? First, change may be imposed from without. For example, the state of Texas required Texas medical schools to institute a required family medicine clerkship beginning in 1990. Second, methods of financial support for outpatient teaching may be identified. This may, as in the past, initially come from private foundations or it may come from changes in the way that medical care is financed. Third, medical schools may independently recognize outpatient care as an objective and alter their financing arrangements and faculty reward systems accordingly. It is difficult to predict whether any of these possibilities will become generally operative in the near future.

In summary, the outpatient setting represents a necessary educational supplement to inpatient hospital care for the comprehensive clinical education of medical students. During the twentieth century, there has been some dissatisfaction with the types of outpatient teaching that have been attempted. While the topic is currently the subject of lively discussion, the amount of outpatient teaching that actually occurs is variable and the quality of the educational experiences generally has not been evaluated. A first step should be the definition of objectives for outpatient teaching, and the selection of appropriate sites for meeting such objectives. Once a clear program has been developed, mechanisms to fund the experiences should be explored and strategies to overcome any organizational barriers should be identified.

10

The Medical Curriculum: Developments and Directions

DeWitt C. Baldwin, Jr.

Innovations in medical education take many forms and arise for a variety of reasons. In general, there have been three stimuli for change in the medical curriculum: 1) the medical profession; 2) the social and economic environment of medicine; and 3) changes in the structure and content of medicine, including the impact of new scientific knowledge and technology.

FORCES AFFECTING MEDICAL EDUCATION FROM WITHIN MEDICINE

Pressures for change from inside medicine most frequently arise from efforts toward professional evolution and reform.[1] Although these often have been characterized as self-serving by critics of medicine,[2] proponents prefer to see them as standard-setting and self-regulating.[3] Certainly, the early efforts of the American Medical Association's (AMA) Council on Medical Education (CME), along with the "Flexner Report" of 1910,[4] must be viewed as landmarks in setting the form and standards of medical education in this country. However, although these efforts served admirably to bring a certain needed order, the net result of the "Flexner Report" was to establish both an organizational form, based on the Johns Hopkins model, and a particular emphasis, the life sciences, as the foundations for modern medical education. While this reform effort appeared to arise largely from within the profession, external forces were involved as well.[5]

Perhaps the most important and ongoing effort of medicine to set and insure high standards in the profession involves the accreditation activities of the Liaison Committee on Medical Education (LCME) and the Accreditation Council for Graduate Medical Education (ACGME). Both bodies derive their mandate and support from their parent professional organizations. The LCME has representation from the AAMC and the AMA; the ACGME has representation from the AMA, the AAMC, the American Hospital Association (AHA), the American Board of Medical Specialties (ABMS), and the Council on Medical Specialty Societies (CMSS). Through the mechanisms of periodic review and site visits to medical schools and to graduate training programs, a constant and uniform standard of quality in curriculum and training is maintained. Such professional oversight mechanisms do not exist in other parts of the world, where review of educational programs frequently is the responsibility of governmental agencies and designed to serve national goals.

Licensing of physicians by the individual states, usually by a board of professional examiners, represents another effort of the profession to set standards. In addition, all specialties set requirements which must be met in order to qualify for certification. More recently some specialities have proposed or mandated standards for recertification.

Such efforts from within the profession to guide and direct medical education have continued unabated through the years. Indeed, major reviews of the curriculum have appeared nearly every decade since the 1930s.[6] Among the most recent have been the AMA's "Future Directions for Medical Education" in 1982, and the AAMC's "Physicians for the Twenty-First Century" in 1984, as well as Macy Foundation reports.[7]

EXTERNAL FORCES INFLUENCING MEDICAL EDUCATION

Legislation Affecting Physician Supply

Forces from outside medicine affecting medical education often emanate from social and community concerns about the nature of the profession and its efforts to expand, contract, regulate, or empower itself. Frequently this social concern is translated into legislation. One area of legislation that profoundly influenced medical education in the 1960s and 1970s was the federal attempt to increase the number of physicians, exemplified by the passage of the Health Professions Educational Assistance Act of 1963 and the Health Manpower Act of 1968. These two acts provided the stimulus and, perhaps more important, the funding that led to the creation of some thirty-eight new medical schools between 1960 and 1985, along with a doubling of the number of medical students.[8]

While the intent of this legislation was primarily to increase the nation's supply of physicians, the rapid expansion in the number of schools led to an unparalleled burst of experimentation in pedagogy and curriculum. Although many of the new schools followed traditional lines in establishing their curricula, a significant number introduced new forms and methods of education, such as the integrated organ-systems approach to teaching the basic sciences and the community-based focus for clinical education.[9] Another example of outside forces affecting the curriculum is the government support for the development and expansion of particular specialty areas, such as primary care, family medicine, and geriatrics, which are considered to be in short supply.

Changing Patterns of Health Services

Under current pressures for cost-containment, patients in acute care hospitals, where students receive much of their clinical education, are being admitted with more serious illnesses and for shorter stays than previously. This produces greater stress and demands higher levels of competence from health care providers.[10] The role that students can play in such settings is becoming more limited; at the same time they are deprived of experience with the expanded ambulatory practice of medicine. Thus there is a need to increase the amount of clinical teaching outside the tertiary-care hospital. The skills for treating ambulant, functioning patients provide a desirable educational and ethical complement to those of managing seriously ill patients in intensive care units. Medical schools will need to negotiate with or acquire ambulatory care teaching settings so that they can offer such teaching experiences.[11]

The New Practice Environment

Nearly all forms of practice now call for increased attention and accommodation to fiscal and regulatory demands. In addition, new practice arrangements, such as managed care plans, require a thorough understanding of cost-effective medical care. While brief overviews of the health care system often are provided, the curriculum usually does not include in-depth coverage of areas such as health economics or health care policy. Also, students do not gain first-hand experience in settings, such as HMOs, where the nature and style of practice vary from that of the hospital, and the economic incentives differ.

There is some recognition of the importance of these areas. Some medical schools are permitting or even encouraging students to seek combined degree with schools of business or health services management. In addition, administrative medicine is one of the fastest growing specialties of medicine.[12]

The Health Care Team

The increasing complexity of patient care and the broad range of skills needed to manage certain conditions requires an integrated team approach.[13] The concept of multi-disciplinary team care calls for greater interdisciplinary experience on the part of students from all the health professions and particularly those from medicine, who frequently will become the de facto medical decision-makers and leaders of such teams. Ideally, such teamwork and leadership skills should be learned early and continuously throughout professional education. However, most medical education continues to occur in isolation from that of other health professions, even in settings where such contact is possible, such as academic health science centers and hospitals. Medical students generally learn little about the roles and expertise of other health professionals; this makes team work based on mutual understanding and respect difficult.

CHANGES IN THE STRUCTURE AND CONTENT OF MEDICINE

A third set of influences on the medical curriculum are those resulting from changes in the nature and content of medicine itself, including the emergence of new scientific knowledge and technology.

Growth of New Specialties

One important trend has been the increasing specialization within medicine. One by one, new clinical specialties and subspecialties have appeared and separated from the traditional disciplines of medicine and surgery. Pediatrics, for example, acquired a unique clinical and scientific base in the 1920s and early 1930s, becoming established as a recognized specialty with the establishment of the American Board of Pediatrics in 1933.[14]

In similar fashion, psychiatry and neurology gradually emerged from internal medicine and assumed a place in the curriculum. In 1909, the AMA CME recommended a minimum of thirty hours of psychiatry in all medical schools.[15] By 1931–32, psychiatry averaged some seventy-seven hours across a sample of sixty-six schools, 43 percent of which taught an average of sixteen hours of psychiatry at the pre-clinical level.[16] The 1962 Group for the Advancement of Psychiatry report indicated that the pre-clinical teaching of psychiatry had increased to an average of seventy-three hours per school; in 1966 Webster found this average to be ninety-six hours.[17] The American Board of Psychiatry was formed in 1934.[18]

These two examples illustrate the emergence of new clinical disciplines. Each was accompanied by a gradual increase in curriculum time and academic staffing. One effect of such growth in the specialities was a progressive division of the curriculum into smaller units to accommodate students' need for knowledge and experience in each. Thus, the length of most clinical clerkships has been reduced, greatly affecting the nature of the student learning experience.

In the public interest, social and political forces inside and outside medicine have responded to this specialization. For example, the increasing concern over access to health care in the 1960s and early 1970s led to the perceived need for a "primary care physician," which in turn played a key role in the emergence of family practice as a specialty.[19]

New Knowledge and Technology

A related set of forces involves the rapid proliferation of knowledge in science and technology, which has transformed the volume of information and substantive content of both the basic and clinical sciences. Following the "Flexner Report," there emerged a relatively standard curriculum for most medical schools in the United States.[20] This consisted of two years of basic science courses followed by two years of clinical experiences. Neither Flexner nor the other medical educators of his time could have imagined the enormous developments in scientific knowledge, nor the pressures toward specialization which would occur during the twentieth century. As in clinical medicine, the growth of scientific knowledge led to specialization in the basic sciences, which in turn has produced a number of new scientific disciplines, such as cell biology, endocrinology, immunology, and the neurosciences. Each of these, in turn, has added new disciplinary and cross-disciplinary knowledge and methods to the curriculum, including such recent additions as "neuro-psychoimmunology." Integrating the "new biology" has imposed enormous and increasing pressure on the structure and content of the preclinical curriculum.

At the same time, the demand for clinical and social relevance has led to increasing amounts of early clinical and community-based experiences, as well as the addition of content from the social and behavioral sciences, medical humanities, and ethics to the first two years of the curriculum.

The rapid development and expanded use of new technology affects the learning environment as well as patient care. Students must learn to use and depend upon such technologies, sometimes to the detriment of more traditional clinical and interpersonal skills. The use of such equipment also limits the settings in which students can work, as well as the level of responsibility they can assume for patient care.

SOME CURRENT AND CONTINUING ISSUES IN THE CURRICULUM

As a result of internal and external forces as well as perceived problems in medical education, a number of curriculum changes have been considered and sometimes implemented. In a number of areas change has not yet occurred, and it is needed.

Length of Medical Education

During the last 150 years, the length of training required for medicine has greatly increased in response to the expanding scientific knowledge base and the demands for quality control. The standard four-year medical curriculum was adopted by the beginning of this century. However, the response to the incredible explosion of scientific knowledge and therapeutic technology since then has been to increase the content of an already over-crowded curriculum without any regard for the process of learning. In order to accommodate this great increase in content, especially in the first two years, the major instructional format has been the lecture.

After a brief experiment with speeding up the curriculum during World War II and with shortening the medical curriculum to three years during the late 1960s and early 1970s, both in response to perceived manpower needs, nearly all medical schools have returned to a four-year program. Most are finding even this too brief a time to teach all the knowledge and skills felt to be required of the modern physician.

Another effort to shorten medical education and relieve the intense pressures of the premedical curriculum has involved combining college and medical education into a shortened six- or seven-year curriculum. Such programs currently exist at twenty-nine medical schools. Apparently they are successful.[21]

Recently, Robert Ebert and Eli Ginzberg have proposed a radical restructuring of medical education.[22] They advocate eliminating or transforming the current fourth year—largely electives in most schools—into a basic internship, thus enabling students to move more rapidly into specialty training. This type of program has been implemented at the University of Kentucky, which has introduced a "three plus three" curriculum track. The first three years of the curriculum lead directly into a three-year residency training program in family medicine or internal medicine. The M.D. degree is granted at the end of four years.

In addition to the content overload in the undergraduate medical curriculum, there has been an increase in the length of graduate medical education in nearly every specialty. Many graduates of the 1940s and 1950s went into practice after a single year of internship, but most physicians today are taking three or more years of graduate education (some as many as eight or nine) to prepare for the demands of modern practice. Indeed, there are constant calls for even longer and more rigorous training programs.

Philosophy and Pedagogy

The question must be raised whether the emphasis for change should focus primarily on desired clinical outcomes and on learning styles or on the length of education and training. Certainly these are not independent. Modern pedagogy provides a number of radically new and different alternatives to memorization and rote learning. Such strategies as problem-based and simulation learning and interactive, computer-assisted instruction appear to better integrate knowledge and application for the student.[23] Furthermore, such techniques may help foster intellectual curiosity, critical thinking, and self-learning, qualities espoused by all educators. Since modern information storage and retrieval technologies have become available, it is no longer necessary for students to memorize vast amounts of content relating to all the disciplines of medicine. Instead, students need to learn how to acquire and synthesize information, and how to apply it. Preparation for the coming "information age" in medicine will require major changes in attitude and pedagogy.

In the 1960s and 1970s, many medical schools introduced new ways of organizing the basic science curriculum, to increase relevance and to enhance learning. The integrated-organ-systems approach adapted from the Case-Western Reserve experience required faculty members from different departments to collaborate in curriculum planning and implementation. Such changes needed strong commitment and expert leadership.

Another innovative aspect of the curriculum at many schools was the early introduction of the student to patients, as well as to community experiences. Once again, Case-Western Reserve was a pioneer in the early 1950s, assigning first-year students to families they were expected to follow throughout medical school. Designed to enhance the relevance of the basic sciences, this experiment, although later altered significantly, influenced many schools to adopt similar programs.

The move towards a community base and orientation has been, in part, a response to the increasing concern and focus on the unmet health needs of the community, as well as the implied failure of medical schools to prepare physicians with experience and interest in meeting the needs of the underserved. However, part of this effort undoubtedly resulted from the reduction in federal support for the construction of large tertiary-care and university teaching hospitals.

Unfortunately, the eventual fate of many of these innovative efforts was a gradual return to the norm of the traditional discipline-oriented, content-based curriculum. This reversion to the traditional can be attributed to many causes: pressure from accrediting agencies, the fact that the "second wave" of medical faculty recruited into new and innovative schools usually came from more traditional schools, and the increasing pressure on faculty to generate income from patient care and research grants. Another powerful factor was that the reward systems of the schools did not recognize the efforts of faculty needed to implement the creative, but often unfamiliar and time-consuming, ideas of the innovators. Thus, many schools have seen innovative ideas and efforts abandoned or severely constrained.

By 1980 it was clear that relatively few schools had been able to preserve the philosophy, form, and spirit of educational innovation that had occurred in the 1960s and 1970s, and that most medical education had returned to "business as usual." Fortunately, some of the innovations have survived, and such features as early clinical experience have been introduced into nearly all schools.

It is now apparent that not only have the impetus and funding for educational innovation declined to the point where few schools can afford to experiment with an entire curriculum, but also the climate and context for change have shifted. The awareness of limited resources and the need for making difficult choices have begun to affect the economy at large and medical education. In this cost-containment environment, large-scale educational experiments and costly faculty-student ratios are difficult to justify, and medical schools have begun to scale back and to look for new sources of revenue to replace the federal subsidies of the past.

Unfortunately, the search for new resources, primarily research grants and patient income from faculty practice plans or significant private practice, has itself profoundly influenced the curriculum, as well as the quality and quantity of teaching. Such demands on faculty time and energy, aided and abetted by the institutional reward systems, have tended to discourage the labor-intensive, small group problem-solving innovations which most reports have recommended, and have reinforced the traditional lecture format. Students universally complain about the lack of personal contact with faculty and there is evidence that even their clinical work is not satisfactorily supervised.[24]

STRUCTURING INNOVATION

Alternative Curriculum Tracks

In this context, a relatively recent approach to innovation has been the creation of an alternative curriculum track within the medical school.

This approach has aroused significant interest in this country and abroad. There have been some examples of innovative tracks that have existed for some time, including the well-established and increasingly emulated Primary Care Curriculum at New Mexico, and Michigan State's focal problem Track II.[25] More recent entries include the Alternative Curriculum at Rush Medical School and the Oliver Wendell Holmes Society Alternate Pathway at Harvard. It is of note that this last "experiment" has now been implemented, in a modified form, as the "regular" curriculum at Harvard.[26] Certainly, at a time when no new medical schools are being planned and the interest in and opportunity for major revisions of the curriculum are severely constrained, the concept of re-apportioning existing resources to create alternative curricular approaches to educating physicians for a rapidly changing world appears to be a significant and worthy effort. Of perhaps even greater significance and relevance is the fact that such efforts are meeting with interest and support in the rest of the world, especially the developing nations, whose needs and resources call for more flexible and adaptive models than traditional medical education in the United States has offered to date.[27]

Another approach to the problem of the "curriculum crunch" in medical education was implemented by Baldwin and his colleagues at the University of Nevada in the late 1960s and early 1970s.[28] In addition to re-orienting basic pre-medical courses in chemistry, biochemistry, and physics toward the life sciences, and introducing human anatomy and physiology, cell biology, and pharmacology at the pre-baccalaureate level, this approach involved displacing some of the content and skills associated with community health and the behavioral sciences downward into a university-based, interdisciplinary, pre-professional curriculum, which included all students enrolled in pre-medicine, pre-dentistry, pre-nursing, pre-medical technology, pre-physical therapy, pre-social work, and pre-pharmacy. These students, taught by an interdisciplinary faculty, participated in a prescribed series of required life science core courses, as well as courses in communication, interviewing, bioethics, health policy, and medical economics. Such a pre-medical curriculum is in line with that recently proposed by leading thinkers.[29]

This curriculum also featured a primary care team experience for pre-professional and professional students in a clinic staffed by an interdisciplinary faculty with advanced health team skills. Students from this background later arrived at their professional schools with a clear base of knowledge and skills in areas often inadequately taught or emphasized in those schools. This experiment clearly recognized the need to educate all health professional students in these important and common areas of knowledge and skill.

Integrating New Content Areas

The explosion of new knowledge and technology in medicine and the need to somehow integrate this content into the medical curriculum has been described. There also is a continuing call for broadening the base of knowledge and skills in the social and behavioral sciences as well as the humanities.[30] Modern medical care requires increased awareness of patient behavior and lifestyle as well as of the ethical and economic dimensions of the problem. Communication skills may be as important as clinical ones for increasing patient compliance and decreasing patient dissatisfaction and malpractice claims.

Somers recently has called attention to four "orphan" content areas currently "neglected" in medical education, all of which appear to be increasingly essential to today's practice of medicine.[31] These subjects are preventive medicine, geriatric medicine, health economics, and medical ethics. Others could be added, all equally important and desirable for today's physician.

The issue of where to place essential new knowledge and skills has plagued not only curriculum committees but also the National Board of Medical Examiners (NBME). Because of the potential impact on curriculum design and content, the NBME has been relatively conservative about accepting new subjects for formal examination. Behavioral Sciences has been one of the most recent additions.[32] At the same time, new knowledge and disciplines are continually entering the field and questions related to these areas tend to be introduced into the most relevant portion of the NBME examinations. Since many of the newer areas represent input from the broad social context of medicine, a number of these subject areas have appeared in the Part I—Behavioral Sciences examination. While meeting a functional need, this is not an entirely desirable development, as it leads to a distortion of the true content of the social and behavioral sciences.

A study primarily aimed at examining the increase in the teaching of the social and behavioral sciences in the medical curriculum from 1972–1973 to 1982–1983 found that a significant number of course titles and a significant amount of curriculum time were devoted to what the authors termed "non-traditional" content categories. These included course titles in behavioral science, human behavior, nutrition, introduction to clinical medicine, medicine and society, and primary care, most of them relatively recent additions to the preclinical curriculum. A total of 669 "non-traditional" titles were identified for 1972–1973 and 868 for 1982–1983. These figures represent 35 percent and 37 percent respectively of the total numbers of course titles for the first two years of medical school.[33]

The largest single area of "non-biomedical" content in the curriculum during the first two years is devoted to "Introduction to Clinical Medicine." While preparation of medical students for their clinical role, by teaching the skills of clinical examination and interviewing, has long been a part of the basic science years, these subjects appear to be occupying an increasing amount of time. Courses in interviewing and patient contact may start during the first year of medical school and students frequently have clinical assignments during the first two years. What is more surprising is that a number of clinical disciplines also are now being taught during the first two years, including family medicine, radiology, and emergency medicine. Curriculum time occupied by these subjects has not resulted in corresponding decreases in the amount of basic science content taught. Rather, the effect has been additive, increasing the subject load upon the medical student. Whether the movement of clinical subjects into the pre-clinical years is due to a subtle pressure to downgrade or de-emphasize the basic sciences or to the increasing power of the clinical sciences or to pressures for clinical or social relevance is not entirely clear. It seems likely that the nature of the subject material (new content), as well as the organization of the curriculum—students remain together during the basic science years instead of dispersing to numerous clinical sites—influences the placement.

Teaching in Ambulatory Settings

More than ten years after Rogers advocated moving more clinical teaching into the ambulatory care setting, most faculties are still talking about whether it is feasible and, if so, how to do it.[34] Much of the infrastructure is there, arising largely from the desire of academic medical centers to accrue referral sources for their tertiary-care services. Indeed, one of the most interesting phenomena of the last decade has been the enormous increase in the numbers of clinical faculty employed by medical schools and/or academic health centers. Many of these faculty members are located in community hospitals, ambulatory care facilities, specialty clinics, and affiliated residency programs, thinly disguised as feeders for the medical center.

With the exception of family medicine, there is little evidence of greatly increased use of ambulatory clinics and populations in the training of most specialties. Even General Internal Medicine and General Pediatric clerkships and residencies do not provide an overabundance of such training experiences, although recent changes in the accreditation standards for pediatrics and internal medicine suggest a move in this direction. Given the continuing power and influence of categorical research funding and the fiscal survival needs of tertiary-care hospitals, it is relatively unlikely that control over the clinical training experiences of medical schools and residencies will soon be relinquished.

The Place of Morality and Medical Ethics

There is a perceived breakdown in ethics in the larger society, and major figures and institutions in business, science, politics, and religion have been tainted with moral or ethical misdeeds. This raises the question how ethics and morality are taught and how they influence the professionalization and performance of the physician.[35] Sheehan and colleagues have reported that the level of moral reasoning is significantly correlated with clinical competence.[36] There are concerns over how students acquire their own professional ethics and standards. Coupled with this are similar concerns about the increasing number and complexity of ethical decisions being forced upon the physician by the growth of science and technology. It is important to distinguish between these two ethical foci in terms of education and curriculum, although at some level they would appear to be inextricably related. Most schools now offer courses in medical ethics and some have experts in this field. At the same time, the length, content, and method of such courses leave much to be desired. These are not purely cognitive, or knowledge-based, fields of study, nor are they best taught in the lecture format.[37]

Medical education, especially in the clinical setting, provides an ideal environment for learning the skills of moral reasoning and ethical decision-making. These appear to develop best in small group interaction around real-life issues, where students are able to exchange views and test values under the tutelage of experienced clinicians and ethicists.[38]

Professional and scientific ethics are best learned in response to real situations. To focus on the teaching of biomedical ethics as something external to the physician's own ethical and moral behavior seems inexcusably blind.

Student Assessment and Evaluation

Student evaluation remains one of the least studied and least satisfactory aspects of the curriculum. As in other educational programs, there has been little satisfactory definition of the desired outcome, the product, the medical educational program is intended to produce. Furthermore, effective methods for assessing non-cognitive elements, such as skills and attitudes, are just beginning to emerge. Indeed, evaluations are still largely focused on competence, rather than the more relevant and germane area of performance. As a result, most schools rely heavily on standard but limited cognitive criteria, such as scores on multiple-choice examinations.

There have been pleas for closer supervision to determine students' strengths and weaknesses. Evaluations based on such supervision would enhance the confidence of the faculty, the profession, and the public.

Significant efforts to improve the learning and assessment of students' clinical and problem-solving skills have been recorded recently by Stillman and colleagues and by Barrows and colleagues.[39] The former developed standardized methods of assessing skills of students in their clinical years; the latter introduced a three-day assessment of senior medical students at Southern Illinois University Medical School, using standardized patients, who help to evaluate the student's clinical and social skills and performance. In addition, computer programs, using an interactive format, have been developed around patient-management problems. These offer a less labor-intensive but still expensive method of evaluation that holds considerable promise for the future, if the financial and logistical problems can be solved.

Among the most intriguing and promising attempts to tie student learning to competence and performance has been the one conducted by Small and his associates at the University of Florida School of Medicine.[40] Utilizing a small-group, cooperative-learning format in a first-year immunology course, he has shown that peer evaluations of students' ability and willingness to help others are highly correlated with fourth-year assessments of clinical performance. These evaluations can be useful in the formulation of Deans' Letters and in residency selection.

CONCLUSION

It is not sufficient, or perhaps even appropriate, to look at reform of the medical school curriculum in isolation. Nor is it enough to eliminate redundancies and overload. The appropriate way to deal with needed changes in the medical school curriculum must include consideration of the interfaces between premedical education and medical school, and between the latter and graduate medical training. Indeed, Todd and others have pointed out that continuing education offers the longest, most promising and needed area of professional education for the future.[41] Ebert and Ginzberg have written of the need to treat medical education as a continuum and have suggested breaking down the walls between college and medical school, much as is done at Oxford and Cambridge.[42]

Despite the many innovations that have been introduced and the fairly constant phenomenon of curriculum change, it seems clear that much change results from shifts in popular fashion and represents fairly minor tinkering with the curriculum. Indeed, the curricula of American medical schools are surprisingly similar and relatively resistant to major revision. Despite many conferences and reports, significant change and restructuring of the curriculum have not occurred and seem unlikely to do so. Among the many barriers to curriculum change is the associated need for required changes in governance, financing, and reward systems.[43]

For significant change to occur and be maintained, certain fundamental issues need to be confronted. First, there is the need for more effective communication and coordination among the basic science departments, as well as among clinical disciplines, to eliminate redundancies and to focus on what is truly essential to the practice of medicine and the education of medical students. This may mean cutting back on the rich diet of scientific exotica derived from faculty research interests and more appropriately reserved for graduate students or those with special interests in academic medicine.

Another important issue for medical education to acknowledge and confront is that not all students prefer to learn in the same way. Apart from a few schools such as Michigan State, Rush, and New Mexico, where students are officially allowed to choose curriculum tracks suited to their individual learning styles, most curricula feature one basic approach to learning (memorization) and one major method of evaluation (multiple-choice examinations). This continues in spite of evidence that these methods are not the most effective, even for the majority of students. Paradoxically, those schools which have attempted to move primarily to a more educationally desirable, problem-solving format may equally disadvantage those who learn best by lecture. Medical education seems to be obsessed with the idea that there is one (best) way of teaching medicine, thus creating a Procrustean bed," which forces students with diverse goals, interests and learning styles to conform or be cast out.

An issue that remains unresolved is whether medical education should focus on the science or the art of medicine. Judging from appearances, most medical school faculties are committed to the former. Science serves medicine exceedingly well where there are linear, closed systems; unitary causes and cures; and predictive probabilities. It often fails to provide much comfort or insight to the individual doctor and patient when they seek to apply these generalities to the idiosyncrasies of a specific condition or encounter in time. Nor does the scientific approach based on disease hold up well around recent concerns with health and enhanced function. Both the science and art of medicine can and must be integrated and taught as such.

Finally, as long as faculty are organized into self-contained, self-sufficient, often self-interested departments which answer to no authority and exist to defend their curriculum turf, needed changes and the prerequisite spirit of communication and collaboration will not happen. In schools where major restructuring of a pre-existing curriculum has occurred, a superordinate faculty body was created to regulate and oversee the process. Most studies of the change process also identify the need for a forceful leader, general acceptance of a new philosophy or vision, and creating of a reward system to match the goals.[44]

To the forces identified at the beginning of this chapter must be added the one which encompasses and overrides all the rest, the public. The demand for a more personal and humanitarian physician will not be mollified by minor curriculum tinkering or a few elective courses. Nor will the student continue to willingly and uncomplainingly accept an educational experience described by most as lacking in sensitivity, supervision, and personal contact.[45] Despite its many successes, something is basically wrong at the heart of the curriculum and needs to be corrected. This problem is in large part a result of the assumption that students are empty vessels waiting to be filled up with facts, and that they all need to think alike and act alike. Perhaps the greatest salvation of medical education has been the diversity of applicants and the independent spirit of some students, who may appear to conform on the surface, but somehow maintain their individuality of mind and spirit. That many do not is unfortunate.

In the end, however, one must remember that the formal curriculum is not the real or only issue. Perhaps most of what we honor in good physicians is learned from mentors, peers and patients, through the so-called informal curriculum. Especially lacking today seems to be the informal, personal contact and role modeling which has characterized medical learning for centuries. Busy residents and clinicians, heeding the call of reward and advancement, are too seldom found alongside the student at the bench or at the bedside. It is not the subject matter of the sciences that de-humanizes, nor do the humanities humanize. It is the nature and effect of the teacher-student relationship that enables the student to integrate the art and science of medicine and to become the complete physician. As Rappleye said in 1932, "the student and the teacher, not the curriculum, are the crucial elements in the education program."[46]

11

Will the Supply and Distribution of Physicians be Appropriate for the National Needs in the Year 2000?

David A. Kindig and Hormoz Movassaghi

Abraham Flexner, writing at a time of perceived physician oversupply, proposed a plan for reducing the physician surplus by decreasing the number of medical schools. His methods of analysis of both supply and demand were far simpler than those used currently. There are, however, some parallels between the Flexner era and our own, when the issue of physician supply has again become a central one.

The purpose of this chapter is to review the recent literature on physician supply and requirements and to raise questions and offer conclusions about the adequacy of the supply and distribution of physicians in the United States for the coming decades. We will begin with the rationale for and the findings of the most important study of this issue in the previous decade, the 1980 report of the Federal Graduate Medical Education National Advisory Committee (GMENAC). We will then review some of the main critiques of the GMENAC methodology and post-GMENAC trends and studies on overall physician supply; overall physician requirements as determined using biologic need, delegation to non-physician providers, and estimates of productivity; specialty and geographic distribution; and international trends. Finally, we will attempt to draw some conclusions and identify questions that should be important for medical educators, policy makers, and health services researchers in the future.

THE GMENAC REPORT

Clearly the most important policy document of the 1980s in the field of physician supply and distribution is the "Report of the Graduate Medical Education National Advisory Committee to the Secretary, DHSS" published in September of 1980.[1] The most significant result of this report was the projection of an overall physician "surplus" by 1990 and 2000, which stimulated an enormous amount of discussion and some research in this field. It is important to spend some time on the study itself, its methodology, results, and critique; but first the political context of the GMENAC itself must be reviewed.

During the fifteen years from about 1965 until the release of the GMENAC report in 1980, there was considerable activity in addressing issues related to physician supply and distribution. The growth of private health insurance and the passage of Medicare and Medicaid in the mid–1960s led to fears that the demand and financial support for health care and physician services would outstrip the existing supply and that a moderate to severe shortage of physicians would occur. No formal studies of this prediction exist in the literature but federal estimates of an impending shortage of 50,000 physicians were very important in influencing policy at that time.[2] In addition to concern with the overall supply, great emphasis was placed on issues of access to health services for all Americans. Increasing the availability of generalists, as well as physicians for rural and inner-city areas, was high on the priority list of many state and federal policy makers.

Many significant programs and initiatives were undertaken at the state, federal, and local levels. Among the most important were capitation payments and construction funds to medical schools for increasing class size; the development of urban and rural Comprehensive Health Centers out of the initial Office of Economic Opportunity; the establishment of the National Health Service Corps for placing federal health professionals in the urban and rural communities, initially as an alternative to service in the armed forces; federal funding for development of family practice residencies and later for general internal medicine and pediatrics; the establishment of a specialty board for family practice; support for nurse-practitioner and physician's-assistant programs; initiation of Area Health Education Centers; the creation of special programs for the training of minority health professionals; and many state-level approaches for repayment of educational loans to encourage physicians to locate in primarily rural areas. Many medical schools began to develop programs in community medicine and family medicine that were intended to encourage careers in primary care, especially in rural and inner city areas. The American Medical Student Association and the earlier Student Health Organizations played a critical role in organizing such educational experiences prior to their incorporation into the regular medical school curriculum.

There is no question that federal legislation and federal funding had the greatest impact in the area of health personnel development, although a number of reports sponsored by private foundations and professional associations significantly influenced policy-making in this period. It was an exciting time for health policy and programs. Experiments were designed and funded and there was a belief that genuine progress was being made toward achieving the stated goals of increasing the supply of physicians and improving access to care. Political support was largely bipartisan; most of the programs of a domestic social nature began during the Republican presidency of Richard Nixon, with the support of the AMA. This partly reflected the general public support of social programs, legacies of the Kennedy-Johnson era. Also, physician supply and distribution issues were of equal importance to urban Democratic and rural Republican legislators.

The results of these efforts were impressive. The number of entering medical students rose from 8,298 in 1960 to 15,351 in 1975, an increase of 85 percent. Board-certified family physicians began to replace retiring general practitioners and more physicians began to locate in rural and underserved communities. As the increased number of medical graduates entered practice, the number of physicians rose from approximately 246,000 in 1960 to 372,293 in 1975. This corresponded to a change in the physician:population ratio from 134:100,000 to 176:100,000.

In the mid–1970s, there began to be concern about the effectiveness of these policy initiatives and about a possible surplus of physicians. During the congressional debates preceding the enactment of the Health Professions Educational Assistance Act of 1976, this concern and the continued perceived imbalance in the supply of physician generalists and specialists received much attention, resulting in a two-year delay in reauthorization. One of the controversial proposals made at that time was for a regulatory "Certificate of Need" approach to the number of residency training positions. This idea was ultimately rejected as unworkable and excessively regulatory, but provisions were enacted requiring medical schools to assure that 50 percent of their first-year residency positions were in the primary care specialties as a condition for receiving federal funds.

The same legislation created the GMENAC, recognizing the need for collaboration between government and the health professions in determining whether the physician supply and distribution in the United States would be adequate in the future. The overall parent committee was composed of twenty-two members, nineteen from the private sector and three from the public sector. Private sector members included physicians, nurses, hospital administrators, insurance company executives, attorneys, and a health economist.

GMENAC is widely known for its prediction of a physician surplus[3] but the magnitude of both the analytic effort and the research methodology are less fully appreciated.[4] Recognizing the limitations of the previous data bases and modeling approaches, GMENAC decided that refined data and new analytic models were required. The "Physician Supply Projection Model" developed forecasts of future supply based

Figure 11.1
GMENAC Supply Projection Model

```
1978 Baseline

    Supply (374,800)

    by Specialty Corrected

    for Attrition (341,000)

            +

U.S. Graduates

    M.D., D.O., Cotrans &

    MSKP, 1978- 1987 (128,000)   --------------------------    GRADUATE

            +                                                  MEDICAL

Foreign Medical Graduates &                                    EDUCATION

Canadians 1978-1987              ----------------------        MODEL -

(4100/year = 37,000)                                           SPECIALTY

            +                                                  SPECIFIC

Residents' Contribution to

Practitioner Pool in 1990        ----------------------

(84,000 x 0.35 = 30,000)


            EQUALS


PHYSICIAN SUPPLY BY SPECIALTY

(FTE) 1990 (536,000)
```

on existing numbers of physicians corrected by actuarial estimates of the attrition rate to 1990, and additions to supply from U.S. and foreign medical school graduates and residents in training (Figure 11.1). This estimate was informed by a complex new "Graduate Medical Education Model," which predicted numbers of students and residents by ultimate specialty category.[5] Future additions to supply required assumptions about the number of graduates of allopathic and osteopathic schools and

Figure 11.2
Physician Requirements Model

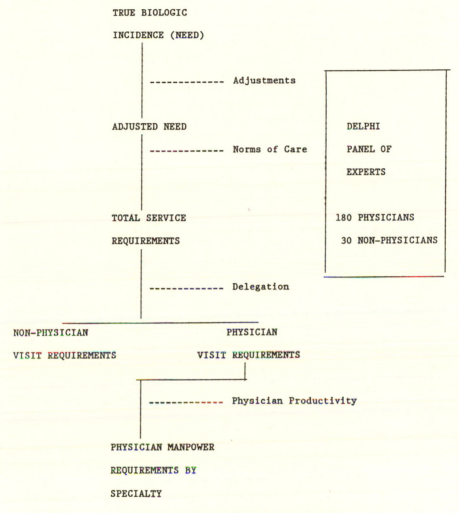

TRUE BIOLOGIC

INCIDENCE (NEED)

------------- Adjustments

ADJUSTED NEED   DELPHI

------------- Norms of Care   PANEL OF

                                       EXPERTS

TOTAL SERVICE   180 PHYSICIANS

REQUIREMENTS   30 NON–PHYSICIANS

------------- Delegation

NON–PHYSICIAN   PHYSICIAN

VISIT REQUIREMENTS   VISIT REQUIREMENTS

------------- Physician Productivity

PHYSICIAN MANPOWER

REQUIREMENTS BY

SPECIALTY

Source: Figures 11.1 and 11.2 are adopted from the Interim Report of the Graduate Medical Education National Advisory Committee.

the number of U.S. and non-citizen foreign medical graduates (FMGs) who would enter practice. Four supply projections were developed, using various assumptions about these numbers.

Rejecting pure need *or* demand-based models, the GMENAC's "Physician Requirements Model" (Figure 11.2) was based on the "adjusted needs" approach, in which estimates of requirements for each specialty were based on assessments of the incidence of each medical condition in the population and the physician services needed for each condition.

Total requirements were based on data and the professional judgment of Delphi panels of physician specialists and others. These panels considered the incidence and prevalence of each disease, norms of care, delegation to non-physician providers, and physician productivity in each specialty. In addition, four technical panels provided information and judgments about the impact of financing graduate medical education, non-physician health care providers, geographic distribution, and the influence of the educational environment. When the supply and requirements projections were compared, there were widely quoted estimates of a "surplus" of 70,000 physicians in 1990 and 145,000 in 2000 based on the "most likely" supply projection. Individual specialties also were examined.

GMENAC reached the following summary conclusions: there will be an overall surplus of physicians in 1990 and 2000; most specialties will have a surplus; the primary care fields of osteopathic general practice, family practice, general internal medicine, and general pediatrics will be in balance, but surpluses could develop for these in the late 1990s; shortages will exist in the specialties of psychiatry, physical medicine and rehabilitation, and emergency medicine; and valid criteria for designating certain geographic areas as underserved were not yet in existence. It should be noted that "surplus" and "shortage" specialties were designated only when supply exceeded or fell short of projected requirements by more than 20 percent. Requirements for the six specialties of neurology, anesthesiology, nuclear medicine, pathology, physical medicine and rehabilitation, and radiology were considered incomplete when the report was released. Subsequent analysis resulted in an upward adjustment of overall physician requirements to 473,000 in 1990 and 506,000 in 2000, with a consequent reduction in the "surplus" to 63,000 and 137,000 respectively.[6]

GMENAC recommended a 17 percent reduction in U.S. medical school enrollment, sharp restrictions on the entry of FMGs, and no further increase in the training of non-physician health care providers. They also stated that: prompt adjustments should be made in the number of residency training positions in specialties with projected surpluses and shortages; the number of minorities in medical schools should be increased; better criteria should be developed for assessing the adequacy of health services in small geographic areas; educational programs should emphasize ambulatory care and training; and changes in health care financing policy should be made that would help achieve these objectives.

POST-GMENAC CRITIQUE, TRENDS, AND PROJECTIONS

In addition to the widespread acceptance by many policy makers and the media of the GMENAC's basic conclusion of a potential surplus of physicians, there has been a large and thoughtful response to the methodology and results by health services researchers. An overview of the general comments on the report and its methodology received by the USDHHS in 1981 is provided by Bowman and Walsh.[7] The earliest substantive critique was offered by Reinhardt in 1981 in his "Alternative View" of the GMENAC forecast.[8] He discussed the GMENAC's need-based approach as opposed to the effective demand forecasting usually used by economists. He questioned whether panels of experts can develop normative standards for health care utilization ten to twenty years in advance, when "there is reasonable hope that future financing and delivery of health care will be rearranged." Thus, the preconditions for effective need-based projections, that is, the ability to translate normative needs into effective demands, may not exist in the current medical care and political climate. While acknowledging the "unprecedented" magnitude of GMENAC's modeling efforts and the value of the advances made in forecasting methodology and data collection, he raised numerous criticisms of the approach. On the supply side, he questioned the validity of the projections related to future physician immigration and specialty practice estimates, even with the new Graduate Medical Education model. On the requirements side, he applauded the use of Delphi panels of practitioners as a way to incorporate the experience of practitioners into the analytic work and asserted that the potential bias or subjectivity of the panels did not detract from this approach. His second general criticism was the predominant use of point estimates instead of ranges for aspects such as substitution of different specialists for specific medical conditions and the delegation of physician tasks to non-physician providers. Mounsey of the American College of Surgeons agreed with the use of the Delphi panels, but asserted that requirements might be overstated since academic and military experts dominated the average practitioner in that process. She also stated that it was hard to accept ten years as a reliable planning period within which there would be no changes in practice setting, case mix, referral practices, and financial barriers to care. She noted that the "delivery system could be seriously crippled by arbitrary decisions based on inadequate data."[9]

Parallel in time with the GMENAC study, the Bureau of Health Professions (BHP) created a separate projection model based on demand rather than need.[10] Market demand-based approaches to physician requirement forecasting, of which the BPH's "adjusted utilization" model was one variant, are largely predicated on current patterns of health services utilization, employment, and productivity, with the assumption that such patterns will largely continue into the future. In the BHP model, the population is divided into eight subgroups characterized by age and sex. The health services utilization of those cohorts in 1980 was used as baseline data, although in certain areas data collected in earlier years were

Table 11.1
The Supply and Characteristics of Active Physicians

	1970	1978	1985
All Physicians	327,861	440,512	538,084
Phys./100,000 Population	163	200	227
Foreign Medical Graduates (Percent of Total)	55,396 (17.6%)	91,070 (21.9%)	114,408 (22.3%)
Women MDs (Percent of Total)	25,507 (8.1%)	42,479 (10.2%)	80,725 (15.6%)
First Year Medical School Enrollments	11,348	16,620	16,929
Foreign Medical Graduate Annual Entry	N/A	4,838	2,738

Source: American Medical Association, *Physician Characteristics & Distribution in the U.S.*, various issues; *JAMA*, medical education issue, various years.

Note: The data on all physicians and physicians per 100,000 population include all MDs and DOs. Information on other components is that of MDs only.

used. In this approach, current utilization patterns are projected into the future based on forecasts of the growth of each cohort. Additional adjustments are made for price, variables such as health insurance payments, and other non-price variables such as change in the incidence of illness and conditions and advances in medical technology. The resulting projections are then translated into specific physician requirements by specialty according to existing employment patterns (such as office as against hospital-based), extent of delegation, and productivity. Unlike GMENAC's "adjusted need" approach, based on professionals' judgment of what level of care or physician services "should be" available, the BHP's methodology specifies what the physician requirements "will be" or "could be" if the present patterns of utilization continue into the future. Interestingly, this approach produced 22 percent higher requirements for 1990 than GMENAC's, with a resulting surplus of 47,000 physicians in 1990 and 78,000 in 2000—considerably lower than the revised GMENAC projections.

Overall Physician Supply

Table 11.1 illustrates the numerical changes in the supply of active physicians between 1970 and 1985. Between those years, the number of active physicians increased by 210,000 (a 64 percent rise). The ratio of physicians per 100,000 population rose from 163 in 1970 to 227 in 1985, as the increase in the number of physicians significantly outpaced the increase in population (64 percent and 18 percent, respectively).

None of the published critiques provide evidence of significant difficulties with the supply side of the GMENAC projections. Iglehart[11] points out that the capacity of the U.S. medical schools has "remained largely untouched" by the political pressure on enrollments. He draws on AAMC data which show only fifteen schools with reductions of greater than five students in the 1986 entering medical school class, for a total decrease of 224 students. Crowley[12] reports that first-year student enrollment for 1986–1987 through 1990–1991 is expected to remain at about 16,200 and the number of graduates to range from 16,300 to 16,600. This is about 2,000 fewer than the GMENAC "most likely" supply model for this period, or an 11 percent reduction in first-year class size. In contrast, GMENAC predicted a 2.5 percent increase in annual enrollment until 1982–1983 and then a leveling off at 18,151. Osteopathic first-year enrollments in 1987–1988 were reported to be 1,692, compared to the 1,868 projected by GMENAC for the mid–1980s.[13]

GMENAC emphasized the importance of the FMG component of aggregate physician supply, noting that the 40,000 to 50,000 new foreign entrants into practice would account for more than half of the projected 1990 surplus of 70,000 physicians. Table 11.1 shows the significant contribution that FMGs have made to the supply of physicians in the United States. In 1970, approximately 55,400 FMGs accounted for 17.6 percent of all active physicians in this country. By 1985, the number of FMGs had risen to nearly 114,408 or 22 percent of the total. While the number of FMGs has continued to increase, the rate of increase has been declining since the early 1980s, primarily due to passage of restrictive legislation. Within the total FMG pool an important development has been the notable increase in the number of United States Foreign Medical Graduates (USFMGs). These are American citizens who receive their medical education abroad and return to the United States for their residency training and practice. The number of USFMGs started to increase in 1970 and this trend gained momentum late in the 1970s and in the early 1980s, increasing from 21,992 in 1971 to 31,961 in 1983. Crowley[14] reported that in 1970, 35 percent of FMGs were U.S. citizens, compared to 55 percent in 1986. While the proportion of USFMGs to all active M.D.s has remained relatively constant, their presence in residency training programs has increased dramatically since 1971, from approximately 6 percent of all FMGs in 1971 to 35 percent in 1983. The overwhelming majority of USFMGs are male; among alien FMGs women constitute more than 20 percent. In 1981, only 45 percent of USFMGs had applied to a U.S. medical school and USFMGs had lower admissions test scores than both accepted and rejected applicants to U.S. schools.[15]

Under the BHP model, FMGs are projected to contribute less to the growth and overall supply of all active physicians in the future then in the previous two decades. While the number of FMGs is predicted to reach 123,200 by the year 2000 based on the "most likely" scenario, they will then comprise about 18 percent of the total supply compared to 21 to 22 percent in the last ten years. Mick[16] has conducted an extensive analysis of FMG supply, distribution, and practice characteristics. He believes that USFMGs retain characteristics from their training which continue to differentiate them from U.S. medical graduates. He also indicates that a decline in residency training positions for FMGs could lead to decreases in physician availability in the North Central region.

No critique of the FMG entry projections is presented in the literature. There were 2,672 first-year residents who were FMGs in September 1985, of whom 1,569 were U.S. citizens and 1,103 were non-citizens. The total number of FMGs in residency training decreased by 828 from 13,337 in 1984 to 12,509 in 1985.[17] It is difficult to compare either of these figures to the GMENAC assumption that 4,100 new FMGs would be entering practice yearly by 1983. There are probably fewer than 4,100 total FMGs entering the practice pool each year, which leads one to suspect that the GMENAC "most likely" supply assumptions may be slightly too high. However, the number of unlicensed FMGs in practice is a potential confounding factor, with 1,210 reported in California alone in 1983.[18]

Although it does not affect the estimate of total supply, GMENAC also expressed concern about the number of minority physicians in the overall physician pool. In 1970, minority physicians constituted about 7 percent of the total, with the majority being black and Filipinos.[19] In 1980, the BHP estimated minorities to make up 11 percent of the total physician supply, with the largest component being Asian-Pacific Islanders. Only 3.4 percent of M.D.s and 1.8 percent of D.O.s were black.

Numbers of minorities in medical schools increased from 7,596 in 1978 to 10,964 in 1985, an increase of 39 percent; however, the percentage of black, Hispanic, and Native American students remains at 11 percent and has not increased despite efforts of the AAMC, and medical schools.[20] Using the BHP forecast, the number of black physicians is projected to increase from an estimated 15,600 in 1985 to 28,500 in 2000. The relative proportion of female black physicians is expected to rise from 26.3 percent of the total in 1975 to 39.3 percent. The supply of Hispanic physicians, on the other hand, is expected to increase more slowly than that of black physicians, primarily as a result of restrictive immigration policies in the late 1970s that have made the entry and practice of Hispanic FMGs more difficult. Overall, the supply of black physicians is projected to increase by 82.7 percent between 1985 and 2000, compared with 34.7 percent for Hispanic physicians. Black physicians will increase from 3 percent to 4 percent of the total by the year 2000, whereas the percentage of Hispanic physicians is going to remain unchanged at around 3.4 percent. Relative to their respective populations, the proportion of black physicians is projected to increase while the physician:population ratio for Hispanic physicians is expected to decline.[21]

Little recent information is available on the specialty and practice location of minority physicians. Keith and colleagues found a larger proportion of 1975 minority graduates chose primary care specialties, practiced in health manpower shortage areas, and served disproportionately more patients of their own racial or ethnic group than their non-minority classmates. Significantly fewer minority graduates (48 percent) were found to be board-certified in 1984 than non-minority graduates (80 percent). These results are consistent with earlier studies which indicated that minorities have tended to choose primary care specialties, to locate their practices in low-income areas, and to serve mostly patients of their own racial or ethnic group.[22] A more focused study of black physicians showed that they are more likely to be in family medicine or general practice and to serve the black population.[23]

Overall Physician Requirements

Both the GMENAC and BHP forecasts project a surplus of physicians, with the BHP model predicting higher requirements, and therefore a lower surplus, than GMENAC. Most of the critiques of the GMENAC report deal with the requirements side of the equation, since this is the aspect requiring the most assumptions in the "adjusted needs" model. Similar assumptions are required in the BHP model but no published critique of these assumptions exists in the literature to date. In this section we will be following the order of the GMENAC requirements model. This approach begins with epidemiologic and professional estimates of the biologic need for services. Then adjustments are made based on assumptions about delegation of certain tasks to non-physician providers. Finally, assumptions about physician productivity enter the model to allow the calculation of the number of FTE physicians required in each specialty. These are added together to arrive at the total number of physicians needed.

Biologic Need and Norms of Care

The first category involves the nature of practice from technological and professional perspectives. Weiner and colleagues and Steinwachs found considerable differences in the diagnosed incidence/prevalence of several selected pediatric conditions in three HMO studies; variations were both lower and higher than GMENAC depending on the condition. Harris cited the cesarean section rate as one example where GMENAC underestimated requirements, since it assumed a rate of 15 percent in 1990. By 1982 the rate was already greater than 19 percent, up from a base of 14 percent in 1978. Similarly the requirements arising from the AIDS epidemic and the increased use of organ transplantation could not have been anticipated in 1978. The nature of the Delphi process also affected the outcomes in individual specialties. For example, whereas the expert panel indicated that 90 percent of the 1.3 million persons with significant psoriasis needed physician care, the modeling panel reduced this to 50 percent. Had this correction not been made, a severe shortage of dermatologists would have been predicted rather than a surplus. Harris argued that most new technology will add to requirements in incremental ways; while the possibility of physician-labor-saving technology exists, he feels that there is no evidence for it at present.[24]

The American Academy of Pediatrics published general criticisms of the requirements approach without going into detailed analyses. They felt that the major assumptions used to derive the requirements figures for child care practitioners were not justified because "the approach understates factors of great importance to child health over the next decade including psychosocial, learning and language disorders, behavioral problems, and the needs of adolescents."[25] It is not stated explicitly, but these commentators appear to be concerned that there may not be an adequate supply of pediatricians in the future. In our opinion, it is not possible to make an assessment of whether requirements estimates are conservative or liberal without a detailed specialty-by-specialty examination of the GMENAC process. Such a review has not yet appeared in the literature.

Delegation to non-physician providers

The next step in the requirements model was to consider delegation of services to non-physician providers, such as nurse-practitioners and physician assistants, in each specialty. The Delphi panel of experts recommended the need for much more research into such delegation and substitution but indicated that until such studies were completed, the delegation levels for 1990 should be 5 percent of normal uncomplicated deliveries, approximately 20 percent of visits for maternity and gynecological care, 16 percent of the pediatric ambulatory case load, and 12 percent of the adult ambulatory case load. They also indicated that the number of individuals training as nurse practitioners, nurse midwives, and physician assistants should remain at 1978 levels. The current and projected availability of these non-physician providers will now be described.

The supply of physician assistants (PAs) has expanded rapidly since the initial establishment of training programs in 1965. At the beginning of 1985, there were a total of 17,000 PAs; between 13,600 and 14,450 were estimated to be clinically active.[26] In 1984, about 65 percent of PAs were working in the specialties of family practice, general internal medicine, emergency medicine, general pediatrics, and obstetrics-gynecology. The relative proportion of PAs in primary care specialties has shown a continuous decline since 1978, according to two surveys conducted in 1981 and 1984. This was primarily due to the decline of PAs in family practice, which still continues to be the most common practice specialty (42.5 percent of PAs in 1984). Surgical specialties employed the second highest number of PAs (18.2 percent), while those in medical subspecialties declined from 6.3 percent of the total in 1978 to 4.8 percent in 1984.[27]

The geographical distribution of PAs mirrors in large part the aggregate distribution of the U.S. population. Some of the states with large numbers of rural and sparsely populated areas such as Alaska, North and South Dakota, and New Mexico had the largest number of PAs per 100,000 population.[28] One study that examined PA distribution by community size between 1974 and 1981 found that the supply of PAs was increasing in the metropolitan areas (more than 250,000 population) and remaining relatively stable in communities of under 10,000. A more recent survey found that 19 percent of PAs practiced in communities of fewer than 10,000 persons. More than half were found in communities under 125,000 population and one-fifth practiced in large urban centers containing more than one million persons.[29] The American Academy of Physicians Assistants projected that the supply of active PAs would reach 20,740 by the end of 1990. This is almost the same as the projection published by GMENAC (20,800) for the same year. No estimate of the requirements for PAs has been published.

In 1977, there were 7,012 nurse-practitioners (NPs) who had graduated from formal training programs, not including those who had only on-the-job training. In 1985, USDHHS reported that there were 26,000 NPs in practice in the United States, including midwives. There are 208 NP training programs with about 2,500 graduates annually. Most graduates have entered primary care specialties. Some are located in rural areas and inner cities but not primarily in underserved areas.[30] The quality of care and patient acceptance have been established for NPs, but there is mixed evidence on their efficiency. This issue will be discussed shortly.

Several studies have commented on the delegation aspect of requirements projections. The most complete analysis is that of Weiner and Steinwachs[31] in the three HMOs mentioned previously. Table 11.2 shows the delegation rates achieved in these HMOs in comparison to the GMENAC "Idealistic" and "Realistic" percentages (the realistic estimates were adjusted downward to reflect estimated 1990 availability). In at least one case, the ideal rates are achievable in actual practice. However, for pediatrics and internal medicine there is an overall 22 percent lower delegation rate, which would result in a corresponding increase in phy-

Table 11.2
Comparison of Overall Ambulatory Visit Delegation Rates at Three HMOs with GMENAC's Rates by Specialty

	Percentage of all Visits Delegated to Nurse Practitioners				
	Normative*			Empirical	
Specialty	GMENAC Delphi "Idealistic"	GMENAC Adjusted "Realistic"	MAX	MCHP	HCHP
Adult Medicine	22	12	15	6	47
General Pediatrics	27	15	0	7	26
Ob–Gyn	43	18	21	41	56
Dermatology	23	18	0	0	60
General Surgery**	–	–	0	0	49
Orthopedic Surgery**	–	–	0	0	44

Source: Steinwachs et al., *New England Journal of Medicine* 314:222, 1986.

*Idealistic normative rates were developed by Delphi panels on a morbidity specific basis. Realistic rates developed by "modeling" panel on overall, non-morbidity basis.

**No explicit rates were developed by GMENAC for these specialties.

sician requirements. The maximum delegation rates were achieved in a staff-model HMO and the lowest in an IPA. The authors state that there are efficiencies in MD-NP teams, but the cost savings may not be passed on in the non-prepaid setting. They conclude that even though NP-PA substitution is professionally acceptable, it may not reach GMENAC-estimated levels because of market forces and decreased supply due to federal training cutbacks.

The American Academy of Pediatrics noted that the surplus of pediatricians projected by GMENAC would be entirely eliminated if delegation was to remain at current levels rather than being increased to 16 percent of the ambulatory caseload. They expressed concern that economic issues may limit the synergism between pediatricians and NPs and cautioned that the role of the NP may be more additive than substitutive. They also predicted that pediatric NPs might be less likely to find "satisfactory practice situations" if there is a serious oversupply of pediatricians and family physicians.[32] Budetti also believed it unlikely that more than the current 5 percent of the pediatric workload would be delegated, even though such care is professionally appropriate, acceptable to patients, and financially lucrative to the practice. This is primarily because of the increased number of family practitioners. However, NPs may still be appropriate to provide service in the rural and urban areas where diffusion of physicians may not have had an impact.[33]

There is little discussion about delegation in the surgical fields but Perry[34] commented that surgical PAs may be one method to reduce the number of general surgeons in training, while still meeting the hospital workloads. Ginzberg made the general observation that physicians are likely to adopt more restrictive stances on NP-PA numbers and scope of practice for economic reasons and also questioned whether the role of these providers is primarily additive rather than substitutive. He predicted that there will be opposition to restrictions on these professionals by their own groups and by the government, which sees them as important for the care of the poor and isolated.[35] Spitzer has asserted that the most important factor in the economic viability of NPs in the United States will be their level of remuneration. Their push for economic parity with primary care physicians will vitiate earlier studies on their cost effectiveness and will, therefore, result in lessened support from government. In the editorial entitled "The Slow Death of a Good Idea," he commented that in Canada the surplus of primary care physicians has all but precluded a legitimate role for NPs in the health system of any province. He was quite pessimistic about the future of these professionals and believed that economics, not acceptance by the public, would be the determining factor in increasing delegation to non-physician providers, or even maintaining current levels.[36] In a more optimistic view of the future, a state nursing association director summarized the evidence on quality and cost-effectiveness of NPs and claimed that geriatrics and long-term care are clinical areas where NPs can make a great difference and will be accepted.[37]

Physician Productivity

Physician productivity is the third component of the GMENAC requirement model. Some estimate of this factor was utilized by each specialty panel to convert physician visit requirements into physician equivalents. Unfortunately, it is not possible to deduce an overall physician productivity measure from GMENAC which could then be compared to 1986 data. Consequently, we will review productivity in three areas: general considerations, the rising number of women physicians, and the impact of prepaid practice.

An extensive review and analysis of physician productivity in relation to supply was carried out by Reinhardt in 1975.[38] He identified four possible areas where increased productivity could be achieved in medical practice: increased number of multi-specialty groups, increased use of capital equipment, increased prepayment, and the increased use of an-cillary personnel. He argued that the use of ancillaries has the most potential and showed that productivity increases of up to 50 percent could be achieved through the use of additional nurses and clerical staff. In his analyses, he did not include PAs and NPs since he used data from 1965. Such productivity increases could be devoted to increased leisure time or to provision of unneeded excess care.

Although written at a time when a physician shortage was still accepted by most policy makers, Reinhardt's basic framework is rich and extensive. He began by noting that the market for physician services and the eco-nomic consequences of excess supply differ from the competitive norm because demand is not independent of supply. This conclusion is based on evidence that physicians work to meet a target income and that they can increase demand marginally, independent of need. He indicated that "base" economic motives do not have to be the reason for increased services: both patients and physicians may agree that resource intensity is related to quality, particularly when reimbursement comes from third-party payers. He believed that an increased supply of physicians will increase, not decrease, the costs of medical care with the consequences borne by consumers and payers. Ginzberg and Davis both agreed with Reinhardt's analysis. Davis estimated that $52 billion would be added to health care costs between 1978 and 1990 as a result of the increased number of physicians. She noted that in areas with more physicians, there were higher medical expenditures for specialists, lower practice expenses due to hiring of fewer ancillary personnel, and physicians saw fewer patients per week. Net incomes were lower in high supply areas, since utilization could not be increased enough, even with increased fees, to maintain income parity. This suggests a limit to the physician-induced-demand hypothesis.[39] Luft and Arno[40] indicated that through 1982, the increased supply of physicians produced no extensive price competition since generally increases were stable, visits per capita were the same, and total services and fees increased.

Unpublished data from AMA socio-economic surveys confirm the pre-dictions of previous writers about the effects of increasing physician supply. Between 1975 and 1987 total weeks practiced per year remained constant. There was a decline in weekly office visits by 1.36 percent per year, weekly hours worked by 0.4 percent per year, and real earnings of 0.05 percent per year, while office visit fees increased by 1.53 percent per year. Declines were greater for young physicians and primary care physicians than for older physicians.

A discussion of the increasing number of women in medicine is in-cluded since female physicians traditionally have been less "productive" than male physicians. Table 11.1 shows that the number of female MDs increased more than three times during the 1970 to 1985 period, raising the percent of women MDs from 8.1 in 1970 to 15.7 in 1985. In 1985, 34 percent of entering students were female, as were 31 percent of the graduates. The number of female physicians is projected to increase, reaching 144,000 by the year 2000. This will be 21 percent of the physician supply.[41] Female physicians are largely found in the five specialties of internal medicine, pediatrics, psychiatry, family practice-general practice, and obstetrics-gynecology. Compared to male MDs, they more often practice in hospital-based or institutional settings, with fixed-salary and regular-hour arrangements and they have lower productivity and tend to practice in urban locations.[42] Based on 1979 data, female physicians work fewer hours per week than males regardless of specialty, with the exception of general practitioners. This was not attributed to child care responsibilities, but to subordination of their careers by married women physicians with high combined family incomes.[43] The lower female physician productivity was projected to reduce the GMENAC surplus in 2000 by 41,000 physician equivalents or 28 percent. This could be a conservative estimate since productivity decreases with age and most women in medicine are below the average physician age.[44] Relman [45] observed that the increasing number of women in medicine may reduce the oversupply of specialists, reduce the projected surplus through lower productivity, and hasten experimentation with alternative arrangements to fee-for-service practice. He commented that women physicians may also have an important influence on national health policy issues, if they are, in fact, more sensitive to social issues than their male colleagues.

The final aspect of this "requirements" section is a review of several demand-based studies which looked at physician requirements in prepaid practice. Weiner and Colleagues[46] discussed the importance of a demand-based methodology rather than a need-based approach. These authors reviewed the historical controversy over using a technical approach to need, independent of an economic analysis of the demand for care. They concluded that GMENAC projected much higher physician requirements than the staffing norm in the HMOs they studied, and that the use of expert opinion in need-based approaches leads to inflated estimates of requirements because of professional idealism. They caution that professionals whose judgments are not independent of their own economic interests should not express such views solely on behalf of patient care and independent of current market forces.

Tarlov took a somewhat more theoretical approach using the same perspective. He argued that the GMENAC adjusted needs model is still appropriate for the fee-for-service system but that a demand-based approach is needed for the pre-paid setting, because of its explosive growth and the built-in controls and incentives in that setting. He proposed the ratio of 120 physicians per 100,000 population as a reasonable estimate of the physician requirement for the 120 million people who will receive their care in pre-paid settings in the year 2000. This would leave 150 million persons in the fee-for-service sector, where he estimated an M.D. per 100,000 ratio of 323, a ratio approximately 2.7 times greater than for pre-paid settings. The concentration of specialists in the fee-for-service sector would be even more substantially "enriched." Unpublished estimates of selected subspecialties indicated possible ten-fold greater ratios in this sector.[47]

One paper has taken the contrary view, claiming that supply and demand will be in approximate balance by the year 2000. The authors project a shortage of 7,000 physicians based on a growth in demand for services of 1.6 percent per person per year. For the supply-side calculations, they excluded 112,000 physicians in non-patient care activities. In this category, they projected increases from 14,000 to 24,000 physicians in administration and from 19,000 to 37,000 physicians in research. They also projected a 15,000 FTE reduction in patient care physicians due to reduced work load of residents. The authors estimated that 75 percent of these reductions will be absorbed by non-physician providers. Finally, they projected that demand 50 percent greater than their estimates could result in a shortage of 60,000 physicians; a demand 50 percent less than their estimates could result in a surplus of 40,000 MDs.[48]

Physician Specialty Distribution

The growth in the total number of physicians has differed widely in various specialties. While the supply of primary care physicians—those with a self-reported primary specialty in family practice, general practice, general internal medicine, or general pediatrics—has grown, the proportion of primary care MDs has remained relatively constant, from 37.7 percent of all professionally active MDs in 1970 to 37.8 percent in 1985. Within the primary care specialties, the decline in the number of general practitioners has been partially offset by the emergence and relatively rapid growth of family practice since 1969. A moderate increase in the number of physicians with specialties of internal medicine and pediatrics also has helped offset the decline in the number of general practitioners, to produce a relatively constant rate of growth in the primary care specialties.

Some authors and studies include obstetrics and gynecology and the subspecialties of internal medicine and pediatrics as primary care. This substantially increases the absolute and percentage values of primary care providers. If these physicians are included in calculations, the fact should always be noted.

It is not clear whether the decision of students who select a primary care residency program will be maintained through graduate medical

Table 11.3
Comparison of 1985 Physician Supply in Selected Specialties with Corresponding GMENAC 1990 Projections

Specialty	1985 Supply	1990 (GMENAC Projections)
General Internal Medicine	58,374	73,800
General/Family Medicine	62,547	64,400
Psychiatry	29,285	30,500
General Surgery	32,252	35,300
Obstetrics/Gynecology	27,865	35,450
Orthopedic Surgery	15,345	20,100

Source: The 1985 figures are calculated by the authors based on GMENAC's Residents FTE methodology and using data reported in AMA's *Physician Characteristics and Distributions in the U.S.*, 1986 Edition.

education, fellowship, and practice. Indeed, if developments of the recent past are any indication of future trends, the prospect of a rising proportion of primary care providers is in doubt. Although 57.5 percent of recent medical school graduates accepted entry level residency positions in primary care, only 31.8 percent eventually entered primary care practice. This varied across specialties. Ninety percent of physicians starting graduate medical education in family practice eventually entered primary care practice, but only 38 percent of those trained in internal medicine practiced general internal medicine. The remaining 62 percent enter the medical subspecialties. This finding was identical to a 62 percent rate of subspecialization in internal medicine reported in a longitudinal study of internal medicine residency and fellowship training.[49]

The number of primary care physicians is forecast to increase by nearly 96,000, a growth rate of 53 percent between 1981 and 2000, with pediatrics leading others with a growth rate of 74 percent, followed by internal medicine with a rate of 59 percent, and finally family practice-general practice at 56 percent.[50] The percentage of primary physicians in the total physician supply, however, is going to increase only slightly. Medical specialties are projected to have the highest rate of growth (74 percent) of any specialty group while surgical specialties are expected to have the lowest (34 percent). There will be wide variations in growth rates across specialties. Since the GMENAC, the shortage specialties have increased residency positions by 7.9 percent and the oversupplied by only 1.0 percent.[51] Table 11.3 illustrates the growth in physician supply for selected specialties. All are growing rapidly. By 1985, some had reached more than 75 percent of the GMENAC 1990 projections. In family practice-general practice and psychiatry, 97 percent and 96 percent of the GMENAC-projected requirements had already been achieved.

The general concern of policy makers has been that the education of physicians has overemphasized the creation of specialists. It has also been argued that the financial incentives for specialty practice, as well as the fact that residency training programs are sized in large part in response to patient care needs of hospital services, have been responsible for this situation. Kindig and Dunham[52] projected that there could be a 55 percent increase (81,000) in primary care physicians and a 111 percent increase (260,000) in specialists by the year 2020 when the overall growth in physician supply reaches a maximum. They suggested that, while it is conceivable that the health care system will be able to absorb the additional primary care physicians, it is more difficult to imagine a need or demand for so many additional specialists. Tarlov[53] is more cautious in his conclusions, simply stating that the fee-for-service sector will demonstrate specialist "enrichment and disparity" in comparison with the pre-paid compartment, and that there will be a declining demand for the time of all physicians. Schwartz and colleagues[54] reported a different conclusion for internal medicine. They asserted that every city of greater than 50,000 needs a board-certified subspecialist in each field and that subspecialists may be warranted in cities from 30,000 to 50,000. Adjusting the projected supply by an amount assumed to represent this increased demand, they concluded that by the year 2000 there will be 7,000 too few medical subspecialists in cities of this size.

Several specialty-specific studies have been published in response to GMENAC. Stern[55] wondered if the projected doubling of the supply of dermatologists would be needed in 2000 with the current static demand for office care, cost-containment efforts, and the growth in the numbers of primary care physicians and plastic surgeons. Kurtzke assumed that neurologists would be primary care physicians for patients with neurologic disease and, therefore, would be in shortage in 2000.[56] In contrast, Menkin and Sheps indicated that only 25 percent of neurologists are primary providers and that there is currently an oversupply.[57] This oversupply has the following consequences: lower quality because of fewer patients per specialist, overuse of technology, higher costs, and deleterious impact on academic centers as fewer complicated patients are referred. The authors reported that fifty percent of a neurologist's workload consists of headache, backache, and epilepsy which could be handled by primary care providers.

According to Schroeder, it is "indisputable that we are training too many internal medicine specialists and also likely too many general internists."[58] He suggested the following: discontinuing substandard training programs, especially those with higher percentages of FMGs; accrediting fellowships; increasing the number of general internal medicine residencies; and tailoring training programs closely to educational and social needs. He suggested looking to surgery for guidance in the latter area. Another report, from the European perspective, illustrated that "underutilized physicians trained in surgical and medical subspecialties have insufficient opportunities to keep their technical skills," thereby increasing the risks of adverse consequences of care. They are forced to do primary care, for which they are not "temperamentally or educationally prepared," to take up "slack" time.[59]

Surgery looked at its physician requirements before GMENAC, with important studies of surgical specialists. One study indicated that the number or surgeons should be reduced and operative productivity increased. The authors, Bloom and Peterson, recommended reimbursement only for board-certified surgeons and for surgical consultants, thus eliminating primary care activities, since these are wasteful and of poor quality. Restricting reimbursement to board-certified surgeons would raise the number of operations each surgeon performed to 300 per year instead of 170. The former figure is similar to that for experienced surgeons in England and Sweden. This change would lower the per capita rate of surgery because of the positive correlation between the number of surgeons and operations, and would save resources. In the short run, reimbursement mechanisms should be used; in the long run, tightened accreditation and licensure should be implemented.[60] Perry and colleagues also cited cost and quality reasons for reducing the number of general surgeons. They maintained that currently acceptable indicators may be reduced due to increased capacity to manage complications, and that very few new procedures are being developed in general surgery. They predicted an excess in the year 2000 even with fewer entering surgical training and suggested replacing some junior residents with PAs.[61] They quoted Moore who said that surgery will "look and feel severely overcrowded ... there is no escaping this fact" as a result of the increase from 22 to 45 surgeons per 100,000 population between 1971 and 2000.[62] The sole dissent to the predictions of oversupply is from the American College of Surgeons, who stated that generalists could not be competent in enough areas to permit a radical cutback in specialists. They suggested limiting the scope of practice of PAs and primary care physicians and were concerned about antitrust implications of the profession's constraining supply.[63]

Geographic Distribution of Physicians

While comparisons of the percentage distribution of physicians in different activity-speciality groups between metropolitan and non-metropolitan areas as aggregate units show little change during the 1970 to 1986 period,[64] several important developments appear to have taken place in the physician supply, availability, and characteristics in communities of various sizes and socio-economic features. Two studies from the RAND Corporation were the first to document an increasing geographical dispersion of physicians between 1960 and 1979, a process that was termed "diffusion." The basic premise in those studies was that physicians in specialties that experienced the largest increase in numbers were more likely to move into geographically less populated areas. This was due to the increasingly competitive and nearly saturated markets for physician services in more urban areas which exerted downward pressures on physicians' incomes, forcing them to locate in other areas. The researchers initially looked at changes in the supply of board-certified specialists in eight specialties practicing in towns ranging in size from 2,500 to greater than 200,000 across 23 states. Findings indicated that the percentage increase in the number of specialists in small towns significantly exceeded that in large cities, although the absolute increase in specialists per 100,000 population was greatest in metropolitan areas.[65] These authors later replicated their methodology to look at changes in the supply and specialty distribution of all active non-federal physicians between 1970 and 1979. They found that medical and surgical specialties had diffused into smaller communities, and by 1979 nearly every town with a population of more than 2,500 had access to a physician.[66] A federal report on the changes in the geographic distribution of primary care physicians, using a different methodology, confirmed that the general process of diffusion was taking place but showed geographical variation in physician availability across metropolitan and non-metropolitan counties of various sizes, particularly for primary care.[67]

In contrast to the above findings, other studies suggest that the diffusion of physicians has been limited to certain geographic areas and specialties. Fruen and Cantwell[68] noted that between 1950 and 1978, despite a rapidly increasingly overall physician supply, there were still wide disparities in the number of physicians per population by type of locale, and that while some diffusion of physicians into small communities was occurring, the growth in physician to population ratio continued to be slowest in counties with populations under 25,000. This finding was confirmed by several state-level studies.[69] In a national study on changing physician supply in rural communities between 1971 and 1981, Right concluded that the exodus of active physicians during the 1970s had wiped out most of the overall gains from new physician inflow, leaving a large number of non-metropolitan communities with constant or falling physician supplies.[70] Even though family and general practitioners have increasingly located in rural communities, distribution has been highly influenced by regional population growth and economic viability.[71]

Another aspect of physician distribution is the presence of wide regional variations. While the RAND studies did not find large enough regional differences in physician location to be of policy concern, a recent study concluded otherwise. Kindig and Movassaghi found that for rural counties with populations under 10,000, wide variations existed in average physician-to-population ratios, which ranged from 31.3 per 100,000 population in Georgia to 86.2 physicians per 100,000 population in California. The percent of osteopathic physicians ranged from zero in North Carolina and Utah to 73.3 percent in Missouri, indicating the importance of this type of physician in the small rural counties of many states. The authors concluded that physician supply was less than adequate in these small counties in thirty-four states. This finding was confirmed by a follow-up survey in which physicians practicing in these counties estimated a need for 1,100 more physicians.[72]

Turning to developments in ten U.S. cities, between 1963 and 1980 there was a decrease in physician availability in poverty compared to non-poverty areas for the groups of physicians studied. The ratio of patient care physicians per 100,000 population had increased by 38 percent in non-poverty areas compared to 21.8 percent in poverty areas. However, office-based primary care physician availability had dropped by 45 percent in the poverty as opposed to 27 percent in the non-poverty areas. The conclusion was that the overall increase in physician supply may not adequately correct geographic and specialty maldistribution in urban areas.[73]

International Comparison of Trends in Physician Supply and Characteristics

The rapid rate of growth in the overall supply and availability of physicians as experienced in the United States is not an isolated phenomenon but has been occurring in many other developed countries and in some developing nations as well. Among the industrialized members of the Organization for Economic Cooperation and Development (OECD) for which information was available, the percentage increase in the number of physicians between 1950 and 1980 ranged from 49 percent in Ireland to 351 percent in Finland. Sweden (326 percent), Australia (209 percent), Spain (203 percent), and Belgium (193 percent) were among the high-growth countries. With the exception of Ireland, the supply of physicians had more than doubled in the countries of the OECD during this period. The percentage increase in physicians per 100,000 population ranged from 25 percent in New Zealand to 278 percent in Finland, with Sweden (214 percent), Belgium (156 percent), and Spain (127 percent) again ranking high. In level of physician availability, in 1980 the U.S. stood somewhere in the middle with 180 physicians per 100,000 population, while Ireland (130) and Austria (250) comprised the low and high ends of this continuum. For all the industrialized countries, the average number of physicians per 10,000 population rose from 10.2 to 19.6, an increase of 92 percent; in the socialist countries the ratio increased from 6.9 to 19.4, a growth rate of 181 percent. In the middle-income countries the proportion jumped from 2.8 to 7.4, a 164 percent increase. Low-income countries had the smallest rate of growth (29 percent) and an increase of 0.7 to 0.9 physicians per 10,000 population.

Little cross-cultural information is available on such physician characteristics as specialty, sex, board certification, and nationality of origin, and the data that do exist may not be comparable for various reasons. One study comparing the physician supply in the United States and four Western European countries (Belgium, West Germany, the Netherlands, and the United Kingdom) in 1980 found the United States to have the highest percentage of physicians who were specialists (84 percent), followed by the Netherlands (62 percent), Belgium (47 percent), West Germany (46 percent), and the United Kingdom (27 percent). The United Kingdom and the United States had the most FMGs, compared to a range of 2 to 10 percent in other countries. Finally, the percentage of women physicians was lowest in the United States (14 percent) relative to other countries that had between 15 percent (Belgium) and 24 percent (United Kingdom). In some of the Western European countries such as Belgium, Sweden, and France, the perceived or projected physician surplus has led to reductions in medical school class size or specialty training positions.[74]

CONCLUSIONS DRAWN FROM THE LITERATURE

From the previous evidence and studies on the issue of physician supply and distribution over the past decade, can any conclusions be drawn about what the situation will be in the year 2000 and about what policy changes are either needed or possible between now and then? We first will present the views of others regarding the overall picture and then offer some comments and views of our own.

The first area requiring attention is the reliability of projections of physician supply and requirements. Most authors seem to be quite cautious about projections beyond 10 or 15 years. GMENAC made projections in 1978 for 1990 and 2000 and BHP also developed projections for that time span. Reinhardt[75] used illustrations which reached to 2010 to 2020, and Kindig and Dunham[76] referred to a peak in the physician to population ratio in approximately 2015. However, most authors are appropriately cautious given the poor prediction experience of the past twenty years. It must be remembered that as recently as the early 1970s a physician shortage was considered one of the most important health problems of the country. In 1968, the AMA and AAMC jointly stated that increasing the production of physicians was the highest priority for federal funding to academic health centers. The fact that capitation grants for medical school expansion were not discontinued until 1975 indicates how recently a shortage, rather than a possible surplus, was the primary concern.

Thinking about an appropriate time frame for projections has to take into account the time required for changes in supply and requirements. The very long time needed for an increase or decrease in first-year medical school class size to affect the overall pool of practitioners is a result of the total length (seven to twelve years) of medical school, residency, and fellowship training. Medical schools made an incredibly fast adjustment in the number of first-year students, from 9,000 in 1965 to more than 18,000 in 1982. However, the impact of this increase in numbers of trainees will not be fully reflected in the practice pool until the first or second decade of the twenty-first century. Foreign medical graduates are a component of supply that can change more quickly. A similarly rapid adjustment can be made for PAs and NPs, since their training period is considerably shorter than that of physicians.

Whereas the supply side has a long adjustment period, the demand and requirements factors can probably change more rapidly, as demonstrated by physician requirements in the pre-paid setting. The potentially more rapid changes in requirements, as opposed to supply, increase the possibility of an imbalance greater than if both factors had similar response times. Given this situation, it would seem that the minimum action required should be a careful monitoring of supply and requirements data accompanied by periodic analytic studies, so that the best possible information is made available to public and private sector organizations. The current Council on Graduate Medical Education is attempting to fill this role, but limited support for studies and data collection constrains its effectiveness.

There are several thoughtful and important commentaries in the recent literature on the overall balance of supply and requirements. The first is that of Tarlov, the chair of the GMENAC committee, in his Shattuck lecture in 1983. After reviewing historic trends and commenting on the criticisms of GMENAC and other projection methodologies, he stated that the 1990 projection of 215 physician per 100,000 is judged by most students of this problem to exceed the need and indicated that this would raise the per capita cost of health care. He then reviewed the changes taking place in the industrialization of medicine and in public expectations of health services. Prevention of death and correction of "physiologically measurable abnormalities" will cease to be the principal medical challenge in the future and "the outcomes of medical services of greatest interest to the patient and society relate to the patient's ability to function at a high level in personal activities." The outcome measures of improved patient functioning per unit cost of care will be highlighted by patients and purchasers in the future. With regard to physician preferences in a period of expanding supply, the trend toward salaried positions will continue and young physicians will be willing to trade income for "regular hours, protection from the most demanding aspects of practice, fast startup at no personal expense, ensured salary, and protection from competition." He predicted that this aggregation into organizations will encourage physicians to sacrifice some professional autonomy for collective interests and that collective bargaining with management corporations will become common. There will be more effective pressure from the practice world on medical centers to adjust enrollment and training programs to meet more circumscribed needs instead of letting the service needs of teaching hospitals determine the number of physicians entering a given specialty. He recommended that the growth in the number of physicians should be restrained, since the increased supply will not reduce expenditures and a "demoralized profession will be beneficial to no one." To achieve these ends, he suggested the following policy steps: reduce first-year medical school enrollments to 16,000, increase minority enrollments, restrict future licensure to the graduates of U.S. and Canadian schools in order to discourage U.S. citizens from studying in foreign schools, restrict the entry of alien FMGs to no more than 1,500 under the family preference citizenship clause, and develop a national health manpower policy. He concluded that the current physician supply situation is the "unintended, unanticipated, and an undesirable consequence" of a previous social consensus that more physicians were needed. He believes, however, that such policy changes are "generally forceful and rarely reversed at least in the near term."[77]

Harris[78] commented that an upside error in physician supply benefits consumers and a downside error benefits physicians. He wondered if we need a small standby pool of physicians for "rationing disasters." He argued that the training of more physicians requires more academic programs and, therefore, might result in increases in beneficial research. While physician-induced demand may not be excessive and unnecessary, he worried about reduced quality resulting from reduced volume. He was not as concerned as some that there will be an unmanageable surplus and urged policy moderation to remove only a fraction of the excess by keeping class size at current levels and containing the growth in graduate medical education support rather than eliminating it. He suggested conducting more research on MD incomes, geographic distribution, and introduction of new technology and procedures.

In 1983, Ginzberg[79] stated that a new physician supply policy was needed because an increase in physicians would not reduce costs or improve access, but physician-induced demand would increase utilization and fees without improving the access to care of poor and minorities. In 1986 he commented more extensively on the politics of change in physician supply policies. He stated that some still believe expansion and an excess supply are beneficial because they promote cost and quality competition, and facilitate desired recruitment by new delivery systems, and the easier entry of minorities and women into the profession. On the other hand, contraction is supported by practitioners with declining patient loads and sophisticated payers who believe that cost control requires fewer physicians. The critical question is whether the demand for medical education will decline in the future in response to demographic changes, increasing costs, and altered career prospects. He cites several factors which will make contracting the educational pipeline difficult. First, the current expanded supply will not produce a significant reduction in the number of medical school candidates, since expected physician incomes are still good. Second, there is no evidence that state or local governments are cutting back significantly on support for medical education, since these governments respond to the public and to the principal interest groups. Faculties and residency program directors will not move to cut budgets. While the need for residency positions to meet service needs in hospitals could be reduced with effective use of other health workers, a major problem with this suggestion is that the number of residency positions is now equivalent to the number of U.S. medical school graduates plus USFMGs. Further reduction in residency positions would mean that some U.S. graduates would not be able to obtain training positions, a highly unlikely outcome. Although there have been limited calls for cutbacks from the practicing medical profession, Ginzberg wonders how long it will be before the state and county medical societies recommend decreasing enrollments or closure of schools. However, parents of USFMGs, minority interests, most competitive organizations, the aged and the rural public will not support contraction of physician supply in the near future. He concluded that it took fifteen years to get a social consensus for expansion and that it will not be until the mid–1990s that practitioners facing competition and sophisticated third-party payers will force the issue in state and federal legislatures. An early shift is not likely "not because it is not indicated but because the political and economic muscle is lacking."[80]

Iglehart[81] basically agreed with Ginzberg's political analysis. He cited evidence of recent changes in professional organizations' positions on this issue. He contrasts the 1985 AMA position—that there is no physician surplus and that competition is beneficial—to their 1986 position that extensive analysis of manpower issues is needed. He described the AMA concern about possible antitrust implications of collaborative action to restrict supply, but also reported that some state medical societies, such as in California, are already officially stating that there are surpluses in their states. Iglehart also reported on legislative resistance to terminating residency support for FMGs under Medicare by representatives from urban areas whose hospitals are dependent on such staffing. For example, in twenty-four New York hospitals at least 40 percent of the residents are FMGs, and in eleven FMGs make up more than 80 percent of house staff.

In reflecting on the European situation, Schroeder saw a number of implications for the United States. He was not certain that there would be an oversupply compared to several European countries. That is, the 1990 physician to population supply projection for Belgium was 340 per 100,000 population, for West Germany 326, for the United States 243, and for Britain 171. The dispersed U.S. population might need a relatively higher physician supply. If reduction in supply is indicated, he believes it should come from FMGs, not from U.S. medical school enrollment since we have a lower number of students to population than these European countries. The difference between the high and low GMENAC projections for FMG entry (4,100 as opposed to 1,350) is the equivalent of eighteen medical school classes of 150 students each, so manipulating this compartment of supply could have a sizable impact. He does, however, recognize that such reductions would impact primarily on USFMGs. Schroeder does not equivocate on the supply of specialists, calling it the most significant issue and concern. In 1980 the proportion of specialists was highest in the United States, as compared to the European countries he studied. He urges that the number of specialists should be reduced before addressing the overall number of physicians. Existing methods of accreditation, licensure, and specialty certification, as well as specialty payment rates, can be used to make these adjustments. He concluded that it is not clear whether there will be too many physicians but there will certainly be the wrong mix of generalists and specialists.[82]

Luft and Arno[83] commented that some specialists will continue to do very well but others will be forced to leave the field because of low workload and associated quality and malpractice problems. Specialists may continue to serve lower supply areas but primary care gatekeepers may find lower cost and higher quality specialty services in high-volume urban settings. Physician's accessibility and style of practice including such things as house calls, longer time with patients, and less waiting time may become important competitive factors. Substitution of nurses and other non-physician providers may be limited because the excess of physicians will force down their wages.

Jacobs and Mott reported that HMOs are employing increasing numbers of primary care physicians. The most important characteristics they look for are board eligibility, motivation, bedside manner, adaption to a changing environment, the ability to work in a team with non-physician staff members, and training in U.S. medical schools. The demand for family practice graduates in HMOs is widely reported by residency training programs.[84]

Tarlov[85] sees a steady decline in the demand for physicians' time, citing a 12 percent decrease in visits per week from 1982 to 1984. He comments that increased time does encourage innovation and competition, and could result in more time with each patient, more time for teaching, more time for free care of poor, more time for continuing education, and more time for leisure.

Some authors argue that a physician surplus will not develop. As a result of increased demand and declining production, another shortage could emerge in the first two decades of the twenty-first century.[86]

VIEWS OF THE FUTURE

With all of the historic difficulties in making predictions about projections of physician supply and requirements, we will still attempt to summarize our perception of the recent literature and offer some views of what the future may hold.

With regard to the projection of overall surplus, we agree with those who maintain that a dramatic surplus resulting in significant numbers of unemployed or underemployed physicians may not be likely. Among the requirements which may not have been adequately considered by those predicting a surplus are the impact of the increasing number of women in the work force, the resistance to delegation to non-physician providers, and the increase in employed physicians with fewer hours per week in practice. This view obviously assumes women physicians in the future will continue their traditional lower productivity. It also assumes that major increases in demand resulting from new financing programs like universal health insurance and new technology do not occur. On the supply side, medical school enrollments may decline in the next decade in response to competitive pressures in medical practice and this may bring domestic enrollments into some balance, although such adjustments will not be realized into the next century. Attention must be paid to physicians not in active patient care, and additional studies on trends of physicians in management and research are needed. Also needed is an examination of physicians listed as "inactive" by the AMA, since physicians practicing less than 20 hours per week are included in this category. At this writing many organizations such as HMOs in California and some attractive group practices in the Midwest are having considerable difficulty recruiting physicians. Speculation exists that many physicians are opting for greater financial rewards in the fee-for-service sector, as long as these opportunities exist. It is not clear whether these anecdotes represent lasting or simply temporary adjustments.

The FMG component seems to be the supply category in greatest question, and it has a shorter response time in terms of changing the overall size of the MD pool. The "eighteen classes" of Schroeder is a very impressive figure given the difficulty in implementing domestic class size reduction. There is no need for U.S. students who cannot be trained in the United States to go outside the country for often inferior education. Policies restricting future licensure to graduates of U.S. and Canadian schools should be considered. Louria[87] suggests continuing training opportunities for FMGs while prohibiting licensure. The political power of parents of USFMGs will have to be considered, but with "grandfathering" over time should be manageable. The issue of urban hospital FMG dependence will definitely have to be addressed in other ways, but first it should be determined whether USFMGs are going to these hospitals in the same numbers as their alien counterparts. Demand on these hospitals may fall, since many hospital executives see FMGs as placing their hospitals at a competitive disadvantage.[88] Restrictions on FMGs is one policy decision which could be altered in the future if unexpected shortages develop; and it could be implemented selectively in states with both a large FMG component and a perceived physician excess. FMG entry could also be manipulated for differential ethnic entry if we are unsuccessful in producing enough minority physicians to keep reasonable pace with the U.S. minority populations in the next century.

The evidence that there will be a great imbalance in the number of specialists seems quite convincing from both the domestic and international perspective. The only paper opposing this view is that of Schwartz,[89] which focused only on medical specialists in certain locations. The impact on quality of care provided by underemployed specialists seems to be well supported; the need and appropriateness for specialists to perform primary care is also in serious question. It is very difficult to imagine the fee-for-service sector having almost three times as many per capita physicians (with most of them being specialists) as the pre-paid sector.[90] The arguments for reducing the number of specialty training positions through tighter accrediting and review should be fully explored and implemented. However, it is not possible to do this without looking at the service needs of the training institution, since it is this need which drives the number of residents. Decreases in the length of stay have not reduced the need for staff in hospitals, since intensity is correspondingly increased. However, there is ample room to replace a portion of the first year residents with physician assistants and nurse practitioners, as has already been demonstrated in surgery. The problem here is that a significant reduction in the first-year residency positions will decrease training opportunities for all U.S. graduates. This may be the most convincing argument for the overall reduction in medical school class size, so that a reduction in specialists can be reasonably carried out. Another possibility may be a further substantial increase in the number of primary care training programs at the community level, with limited in-hospital rotations. This would require new relationships between academia and delivery organizations such as HMOs and multi-specialty groups. New educational models, funding possibilities, and faculty development would be required to implement this at a magnitude that would make any difference. In our opinion, the most important incentive to decreasing demand for specialty training would be to equalize the reimbursement levels for specialists and generalists. As long as the present significant differentials exist, the economic incentive to specialize cannot be overcome, particularly among students in substantial debt. The results of the 1988 National Residency Matching Program show that family practice, pediatrics, and internal medicine filled only about 80 percent of available positions. The economic impact of higher-paying specialties, as well as an aversion to treating the large number of AIDS patients in some hospitals, are cited as possible explanations for this result. The efforts to change physician payment levels between specialties, such as examination of relative values by Hsiao,[91] should have the highest urgency and could be the major factor in reducing the burden of excess specialists. Changing reimbursement patterns may also determine whether less complex disease entities are cared for by specialists or primary care physicians. If a shift does not occur, increased numbers of specialists may be "needed" and will be utilized, albeit with reduced efficiency.

The constraining effect on non-physician health providers is one of the most unfortunate consequences of the expanded physician supply. The evidence that these professionals can provide high quality, acceptable, and cost-effective services is complete. It is their competition with physicians that makes these providers the first casualty of the anticipated physician surplus. It must be noted that their cost-effectiveness may decline when their incomes go up and primary care physician incomes decrease. Most economic studies have been done at the primary care level rather than with specialists. Productivity and cost-effectiveness measures should still be very strong for non-physician providers within many specialties. The additional advantage of this group of workers is that the supply can be changed more rapidly if requirements change; and these careers may be more accessible to minorities since the cost and length of training are less. Major efforts to train these practitioners for specialty roles in teaching hospitals and specialty practices should be undertaken, to aid in the reduction of the physician specialty pool and to lower the costs of specialty care.

With regard to geographic distribution, there is some evidence that increased supply is causing physicians to locate in areas which were previously underserved. It does appear, however, that there will continue to be areas so economically and culturally unattractive that special incentives and programs will still be required. For rural areas, eliminating Medicare hospital and physician rural reimbursement differentials or creating an incentive will be useful in some cases. Programs like Community Health Centers, the National Health Service Corps and state loan-forgiveness programs will continue to be necessary for those counties and regions of special need. In urban poverty areas, the continuation of Community Health Centers with salary support for physicians will be the most effective mechanism of meeting these needs, given the number of physicians preferring these areas. Only if some universal coverage for the poor were enacted could private solutions possibly be effective in these needy areas. Similar mechanisms should be tried to reduce the dependence of inner-city hospitals on FMGs so that the political barriers to reducing this source of supply can be overcome.

There is critical need for data collection and health services research in physician supply and requirements. The past has shown the difficulty of making projections, but timely and ongoing data collection and thoughtful analysis of trends can reduce the likelihood of dramatic errors and unwise policy decisions. Both federal and state governments as well as private foundations should support ongoing analytic efforts to understand and trace developments and trends in this field.

12

Abraham Flexner: Lessons from the Past with Applications for the Future

Barbara Barzansky

Between 1904 and 1920, the structure of medical education in the United States changed dramatically. The number of medical schools decreased from 160 to 85 and the number of medical students decreased from 28,142 to 13,798. Those students who were enrolled were better prepared for their medical studies, since the percentage of schools requiring two years of college for admission increased from 2.5 to 92. The increased preparation in science allowed medical schools to eliminate instruction in basic chemistry and physics, and to concentrate on the biomedical sciences. Finally, the general plan of the curriculum moved from passive toward more active learning, with increased laboratory experiences in the basic sciences and hospital-based clinical clerkships.[1]

Abraham Flexner was a central figure in this period of dramatic change in medical education. Indeed, Flexner has come to symbolize the period, and his name has been associated with the curriculum that emerged by its end. Although the chapters in this book demonstrate that Flexner did not act alone, he was a catalyst in a process stimulated by changes in the environment of medicine and medical education. Given the success of Flexner and his contemporaries in transforming medical education, it is legitimate to ask whether the lessons from that period have relevance for individuals attempting to change medical education today. This possibility can be explored by comparing the current perceived problems and forces for change in medical education with those of the early twentieth century.

CHANGE IN THE EARLY TWENTIETH CENTURY

What were the perceived problems to which the early twentieth-century reformers were reacting? Primarily, Flexner believed that the quality of the medical practitioners of the day was extremely variable.

We have indeed in America medical practitioners not inferior to the best elsewhere; but there is probably no other country in the world in which there is so great a distance and so fatal a difference between the best, the average, and the worst.[2]

The "Flexner Report" argued that the existence of inferior practitioners was a function both of the poor pre-medical preparation of medical students and of the ineffective educational experiences to which they were subjected during medical school. Thus, Flexner's recommendations were directed at improving the quality of medical school matriculants and the process of education in order to affect the outcome.

Robert P. Hudson, in his chapter in this volume titled "Abraham Flexner in Historical Perspective," describes these recommendations, which included: (1) reducing the number of medical schools and the number of poorly trained physicians; (2) increasing premedical requirements; (3) "professionalizing" medical school faculty members, through the introduction of a research function and a full-time commitment to the medical school; (4) putting the medical school curriculum on a scientific basis; and (5) extending medical school control over hospitals used for teaching. All the recommendations were implemented to some degree, though not in all cases to the extent desired by Flexner.[3]

Flexner's methodology can be characterized as evaluative. The Report presents a conceptual argument and a model for premedical preparation and for basic science and clinical instruction, and then compares the actual situation to this ideal. In general, the "Flexner Report" resembles an accreditation survey, using methods and criteria similar to those of the 1906 Council on Medical Education review.[4] However, unlike the 1906 survey, Flexner exposed each school's deficiencies to professional and public view.

While the methodology Flexner employed was a definite stimulus for change, other factors were operating which also facilitated reform. One powerful incentive arose from the interaction of professional self-regulating activities (that is, the accreditation of medical schools by professional groups) and the licensing requirements of the states. Flexner recognized the importance of licensing laws as a force for reform when he wrote "The state boards are the instruments through which the reconstruction of medical education will be largely effected."[5] In order to be licensed to practices a physician had to take and pass the examination of a state licensing body. States began to require graduation from a medical school that was rated as acceptable by the Council on Medical Education (CME) of the AMA or by the AAMC for a candidate to be eligible to sit for an examination.[6] By 1920, forty-three of the fifty U.S. licensing boards did not recognize one or more medical schools, so that their graduates were ineligible for licensure. In that year, the eight schools rated in the lowest category by the CME were not recognized by an average of forty licensing boards.[7] Since the standards employed by the CME and AAMC to rate medical schools were based on the new model of medical education, medical schools that did not reform lost students, who realized their future practice opportunities depended upon graduation from an acceptable school.[8]

A second broad factor acting to promote change early in the twentieth century was the financing of medical education. Most medical schools in the nineteenth century were proprietary, run by local practitioners for profit and prestige. Higher pre-medical requirements, the introduction of laboratory teaching, the need for full-time faculty members in the basic sciences, and the required linkages with hospitals for clinical education—all among the standards employed by accreditating bodies—led to increased facility costs and smaller classes. This combination was fatal to many independent proprietary institutions. The institutions that survived found funding sources apart from student tuition. Many became closely integrated with universities, thus a part of the university budget process. In addition, fund-raising activities were initiated, and private philanthropy became an important source of support for some schools. Financial support from state and local sources also became important. All these new revenue sources favored schools that had initiated educational reforms.[9]

A third factor supporting educational change was the shift from the home to the hospital as the major site for care of acutely ill patients and for surgery. The number of hospitals increased rapidly in the early twentieth century.[10] The resulting availability of potential clinical teaching sites was coupled with a recognition on the part of hospitals of the benefits of a medical school affiliation. A teaching mission became more central to the identity of some hospitals, opening up opportunities for medical schools to create the types of linkages advocated by Flexner.

Finally, scientific discoveries relating to the cause of infectious disease led to the introduction of clinical laboratories to improve diagnosis and management and to the need for physicians trained in laboratory techniques. Increasing reliance on the laboratory in practice supported the introduction of this content and these techniques into the medical curriculum.[11] In a "reformed" medical school, students learned and applied the new science both in medical school basic science laboratories and in the ward laboratories of teaching hospitals. The knowledge and techniques acquired in medical school were then transferred into the practitioner's own office laboratory and directly employed in patient care.

In summary, many factors supported the reforms advocated by Flexner and his contemporaries. However, while change did occur in response to external and internal pressures, it did not uniformly sweep across institutions. There continued to be differences among institutions in the details of curricular structure, in resources (including faculty, teaching facilities, and finances), and in student preparation. Despite the differences, a general model of medical education was accepted, based, at least implicitly, on assumptions about educational quality that were the legacy of early twentieth-century reformers.

CURRENT PROPOSALS FOR CHANGE

As in the early twentieth century, the current perceived problems in medical education relate to both process and outcome. The technical abilities and the knowledge of present day U.S. physicians are not an issue, as in Flexner's time. There is, however, concern that medical school graduates are unprepared to fit into the changing health care delivery system and to meet current societal needs and expectations. Again, both pre-medical preparation and the educational process in medical schools are being blamed for the unsatisfactory outcome.

Four significant reports published since 1982 have made recommendations for change in the education of students leading to the M.D. degree. While these were not the only proposals advanced during the past ten years, they have received considerable attention from medical educators.

"Future Directions for Medical Education"

In 1975, the AMA House of Delegates asked the CME to initiate a study of the first year of graduate medical education. The CME decided that the study should be expanded to include the spectrum of undergraduate and graduate medical education. The report "Future Directions for Medical Education" was adopted by the CME in June of 1982. The general theme is

the balance between generalism and specialism required to permit individuals to develop into well-educated physicians who possess a broad perspective of society, extensive knowledge of biomedical sciences, experiences in the several defined areas of clinical medicine, a thorough education in a specialty, and an incentive to continue their professional education throughout their careers.[12]

The authors believe that increases in medical knowledge and technology have had profound effects on medical education, in part through the growth of specialism. The creation of subspecialties has resulted in educational fragmentation, which has acted against broad, general education in medical school. In order to reverse this trend, the report makes recommendations for changes across the continuum of medical education: undergraduate, graduate, and continuing.

This discussion will be concerned with the recommendations related to pre-medical and undergraduate medical education. The recommendations on the preparation for medicine ask that applicants possess a broad background in the arts, humanities, and social sciences, as well as in the biological and physical sciences. Standardized admissions tests, which evaluate cognitive knowledge in the sciences and mathematics, should not be used as the sole criterion for admission. Admissions committees are urged to determine if potential students "possess integrity, as well as the ability to acquire knowledge and skills." There should be improved communication with college counselors, and medical schools should explicitly communicate their requirements and selection methods.

Medical schools themselves were advised to remember that their purpose is to educate physicians, and that they should not assume obligations that would compromise this primary function. The curriculum should "ensure that graduates recognize the diverse nature of disease," and be familiar with comprehensive and preventive care. Students should get a broad, general education—running from primary to tertiary care—with experiences in a variety of clinical settings. "Prudent judgment" should be exercised in revising educational programs "in response to social change and societal needs," in that graduates are "not expected to become experts in all subjects."

Medical school faculty members, the report argued, are responsible for student evaluation and should not rely solely on extramural examinations. Non-cognitive abilities should be evaluated.

Further, medical schools should not rely to excess on a single source of financial support. Too much emphasis on generating income from patient care decreases the incentives to teach and do research.

Finally, volunteer faculty members are considered an important resource. They should have the opportunity to express their viewpoints about the educational program. There should be explicit criteria for faculty appointment and promotion, and the contributions of all faculty members should be reviewed regularly.[13]

"Physicians for the Twenty-First Century," The GPEP Report

Sponsored by the AAMC and supported by foundation funding, this project addressed the general professional education of physicians and the college preparation for medicine. The final report of the project panel, familiarly known as GPEP, recognized that there was "a continuing erosion of general education for physicians" resulting from pressures to which medical education must accommodate. These pressures included: advances in biomedical knowledge and technology leading to increased specialization, increased knowledge about the role of lifestyle factors in health and illness, the trend toward employment of practicing physicians by health care groups serving defined populations, and increased influence of agencies that pay for medical care.

Regardless of these pressures, the 1984 GPEP Report affirmed that "all physicians, regardless of specialty, require a common foundation of knowledge, values, and attitudes." Along with this foundation, physicians should possess a common set of attributes, including caring, compassion, dedication to patients, ethical sensitivity, and moral integrity. The physicians should be "committed to work, to learning, to rationality, to science, and to serving the greater society."[14]

Its authors argued that preliminary education ideally includes "broad study" in the natural sciences, social sciences, and the humanities. Medical schools ought only to require essential courses, giving students flexibility in their premedical curriculum. The Medical College Admission Test should be used only to identify students who "qualify for consideration for admission." Other criteria, such as the ability to learn independently and to develop attitudes and values required for a "caring profession," also are necessary. Communication between medical schools and baccalaureate institutions should be improved.

To fulfill the objectives of a general professional education, the knowledge and skills that students must obtain to prepare for graduate medical education must be identified. Medical faculties should emphasize the development of skills, values, and attitudes to the same extent as the acquisition of knowledge. Health promotion and disease prevention are necessary areas of curricular emphasis. Education should adapt to changing demographics and modifications in the health care delivery system.

The recommendations directed at the medical curriculum stressed the acquisition of independent learning skills by students. Passive learning formats such as lecture should be replaced by instructional modes that promote independent learning and problem-solving abilities. The evaluation methods selected must assess the attainment of these abilities. In the clinical years, medical schools should utilize appropriate settings for instruction and provide adequate supervision. It is necessary to evaluate clinical performance. Electives should contribute to students' general professional education.

In order to facilitate these recommendations, an interdepartmental and interdisciplinary body is needed to develop and monitor the educational program. The educational program should have a defined budget and the support of deans and department heads. Mechanisms are needed to improve the instructional skills of faculty members, who should establish a mentor relationship with medical students.[15]

The Reform of Medical Education

A special supplement to the journal *Health Affairs*, titled "The Case for Medical Education Reform," appeared in the summer of 1988. The lead paper in that issue was authored by Robert Ebert, a former dean of Harvard Medical School, and Eli Ginzberg, a health economist. The authors set the context for their recommendations by describing changes occurring in the health care delivery system. These include: (1) attempts by third-party payers to control health expenditures, (2) increased use of ambulatory settings for patient care, (3) the desire of patients to take an active role in decision-making about their care, (4) the popular interest in prevention and "wellness," (5) the move to use non-physician health care providers where possible in order to decrease costs, (6) the ethical problems raised by the ability of technology to prolong life, and (7) the growing role of the primary care physician in managed care settings in controlling access to specialists. These general changes, the authors suggest, affect how individual physicians practice medicine.

Factors within the educational system also pose challenges. There is a potential oversupply of physicians and a decreasing number of qualified applicants to medical schools. Financial factors include the decreased federal support of medical education, the increased dependence of medical schools on patient care income, and rising tuition levels. The latter has led to increased medical student debt.[16]

Based on this analysis of the context of medical education, the authors propose that the last two years of medical school and the first two years of graduate medical education be combined under the direction of the medical school. This four-year program is meant for students who plan to enter the primary care fields of general internal medicine, pediatrics, or family practice. In order to increase the diversity of educational experiences, medical schools should form consortia to implement this program. Medical schools should identify core faculty, mostly from the primary care specialties, who would take primary responsibility for this curriculum.

The medical schools were urged to adopt more flexible admissions policies, using readiness for medical studies as opposed to years in college as the criterion. Early acceptance and delayed admission programs would facilitate the integration of college and medical school.

To deal with the projected physician surplus and the declining applicant pool, individual medical schools and state governments were asked to examine the size of medical school classes and determine optimal numbers of students. There should be attempts to increase minority representation through support to medical schools with predominantly minority enrollments and through federal, state and private assistance to low-income minority students.[17]

"Clinical Education and the Doctor of Tomorrow"

In 1988, the Josiah Macy, Jr. Foundation sponsored a national seminar on medical education, organized by the New York Academy of Medicine. The theme of the conference was improving the clinical education of medical students. The proceedings were published as a report titled "Clinical Education and the Doctor of Tomorrow."[18]

There was consensus among conference participants that all physicians should possess certain attributes. Among these were the ability to assess the efficacy of medical interventions, skills in the doctor-patient relationship, attention to health promotion and disease prevention, a sense of social responsibility, and the ability to be a life-long learner.

The participants also identified current problems relating to clinical medical education: a lack of consistency in the way health care currently is organized, financed, and delivered; a technically oriented, fragmented educational system instead of a broad system capable of producing an undifferentiated physician; a reward structure in medical schools that gives a low priority to medical student teaching and curriculum development; excessive attention to the results of standardized tests, such as the National Board examinations; and failure to produce socially responsive physicians.

The conference resulted in six recommendations, which the participants felt would help to overcome these problems. The first was to centralize control of curriculum in a unit with authority to plan, evaluate, and revise the educational program. The unit should receive funding to support its activities. This change would enhance the responsibility of the medical school faculty as a whole for the educational program and would reduce fragmentation arising from the current system of departmental control. The second recommendation was to make residency programs the responsibility of the medical school, in order to "consolidate the continuum" of undergraduate and graduate medical education. The third recommendation was to change the reporting of National Board examinations and Medical College Admission Test scores to pass/fail for the former and acceptable/unacceptable for the latter. This would diminish the reliance on these quantitative measures for program evaluation, which may stifle innovation. The change also would increase the use of less quantifiable but equally important evaluation criteria. The fourth recommendation was to move the base of clinical training in certain primary care specialties to the ambulatory care setting.

The fifth recommendation was to require a period of community service at some time during medical education, in order to increase social awareness and responsibility. Finally, medical students should be required to pass comprehensive, performance-based examinations, to ensure basic clinical competence.[19]

Similarities Among Current Proposals

There is a great deal of consistency among the four reports in their descriptions of the forces currently affecting medical education. In general, all agree that changes occurring in the health care delivery system have begun to affect the medical schools and their educational programs. These changes include the methods of financing health care, the modes of health care delivery, the creation of new knowledge and technology, and increased patient expectations. Also, while the report recommendations differ in specificity, emphases, and suggested means of implementation, many of their general goals are similar: ensure appropriate attitudes and values in students and promote diversity in those entering medicine; reduce curricular fragmentation in favor of a broad, general education; increase the priority of the teaching role; and reinforce the continuum of medical education by increasing coordination with preceeding and succeeding educational experiences.

The audience for current reports is the administration and faculty of the medical school. Only "Clinical Education and the Doctor of Tomorrow" additionally directs its recommendations to accrediting bodies, Congress, and national medical education associations. The four reports have been widely circulated, in an attempt to build consensus about the need for change. In the case of "Future Directions" and GPEP, national hearings were held to inform report development. This approach served both to gather information and to raise the awareness of the medical education community about the change initiatives. The implicit assumption behind these reports appears to be that change will arise from within the medical school when administrators and faculty members are informed about current problems and presented with reasonable solutions. There is very little discussion within the reports of strategies by which the recommendations can be implemented, or of ways to identify and overcome potential sources of resistance to change.

The method used by current reformers is exhortative rather than evaluative. Like the "Flexner Report," current reports describe a model of how medical education should function. The "Flexner Report" did not, however, leave medical schools to draw their own conclusions about how well their programs meet the proposed model.

LESSONS FROM THE PAST

Certain forces in the environment of medical education were instrumental in facilitating change in the early twentieth century: licensing requirements, the availability of financial support for "reformed" medical schools, the increasing importance of hospitals as sites of patient care, and the scientific discoveries linked to disease etiology. Are the same general forces now currently acting for or against change?

Licensure

The pathway to licensure used by the majority of U.S. medical school graduates is the three-examination sequence of the National Board of Medical Examiners (NBME).[20] The NBME-Part I examination usually is taken in the second year of medical school, the NBME-Part II examination is taken in the fourth year, and the NBME-Part III examination is taken during residency. In addition to their licensing function, the NBME examinations (mainly Parts I and II) are used by medical schools for internal student assessment and for program evaluation. In 1989, ninety-six of the 127 accredited U.S. medical schools required their students to take and sixty-three schools required their students to pass NBME Part I, which covers content in the basic sciences. Eighty-nine schools used the results of NBME Part I as a measure of the effectiveness of their educational program.[21]

There is a feeling that reliance on NBME examinations (especially Part I) for student and program evaluation hinders innovation. The test is discipline-based and limited to assessing cognitive knowledge. This puts students from schools that organize content differently and emphasize problem-solving skills rather than content acquisition (for example, those schools with a problem-based curriculum) at a disadvantage.[22] Thus, the mechanism used for licensure is perceived to create some of the current problems in medical education, or at least to inhibit needed reform.

In order to be licensed, a U.S. medical school student must graduate from an accredited medical school. In the early twentieth century, the close linkage between accreditation and licensure put the students at inferior medical schools in jeopardy. This was a powerful stimulus for change (or for the disappearance of schools that would or could not reform). Today, there are those who feel that accreditation acts to maintain the traditional model of medical education. For example, the attention that is paid to NBME scores by accrediting bodies may support the discipline-based curriculum model.[23]

Financing

In general, it appears that the current mechanisms for financing medical schools act more to inhibit educational change than to facilitate it. The fastest growing segment of medical school revenue comes from the provision of medical service (38.5 percent of the total in 1987–1988). In addition, federal research funding accounts for about 20 percent of total revenues.[24] Both these revenue sources represent a considerable investment of faculty effort, which is assumed to limit the time available for faculty members to participate in educational activities.[25]

However, there are some positive aspects related to financing. In Flexner's time, and in other periods of significant change (for example, the 1960s and early 1970s), support from private foundations provided the stimulus for innovation. Foundations again are taking a leadership role. In 1989, the W.K. Kellogg Foundation and the Robert Wood Johnson Foundation initiated major programs to support the development of model educational programs. The Kellogg program is directed at using the community as an educational site. The Robert Wood Johnson program includes improving the governance of the educational program and integrating the basic sciences with the clinical disciplines. These funding programs will provide support to a limited number of medical schools, which will then serve as models for other institutions.

Growth of Hospitals (Availability of Sites for Clinical Education)

The increase in the number and distribution of hospitals supported adoption of true clinical teaching in Flexner's time. Currently, the initiative is to move education more into the ambulatory care setting. In parallel with the rise of the hospital as a site for patient care in the early twentieth century is the increased utilization of outpatient settings for health services delivery today. While the sites that could be used for teaching (for example, HMOs, ambulatory surgery clinics) are available, there are problems that must be overcome. A major barrier relates to financing. The presence of trainees decreases efficiency, which results in lost patient income. Other barriers that have been cited include resistance from hospital-based clinical faculty, lack of resources for teaching (for example, space) at ambulatory sites, and lack of patient acceptance.[26] Flexner advocated medical school control of hospitals, but all medical schools could not, or did not choose to, accept this model. As with hospitals, various models of association between medical schools and ambulatory care sites will be needed to incorporate this change into the curriculum.

Growth of Knowledge and Technology

The exponential growth of knowledge in both the basic and clinical sciences has led to the dilemma of what, and how, to teach medical students. As described in other chapters, new content and new disciplines have been added to the curriculum, resulting in curricular condensation and overcrowding. The large amount of information felt to be important has led to the continued utilization of efficient, though passive, instructional formats, such as the lecture. In Flexner's time, most physicians could directly apply the new knowledge and technology to their own practices. This is not the case today. New discoveries have led to the emergence of medical subspecialties and allied health occupations, which claim the knowledge and technology for their own. This technological fragmentation has removed medical students from direct participation in some areas of patient care.

In contrast, other technologies may potentially ameliorate the problems associated with the expanding knowledge base. For example, the introduction of computers into education and practice can help physicians acquire and manage information.

In summary, the forces that facilitated change during the Flexner era do not appear to support current efforts. Financing, with its attendant institutional priorities, is perhaps the greatest barrier. It is hoped that renewed foundation support will allow some medical schools to engage in curricular reform. A note of caution must be raised about this possibility, however. For innovation to succeed, the changes must survive the end of external funding. In addition, if change is meant to be system-wide, medical schools that do not receive funding must identify other sources of support.

Applications for the Future

Given the preceding analysis, is significant change possible? First, it is useful to consider that change may occur at many levels. Within a given medical school there is the possibility for minor curricular revision (for example, adding small group discussions to a particular course or adding a required ambulatory care clerkship) or major curricular revision (such the change to an organ-system-based curriculum at Case-Western Reserve University in the early 1950s). Finally, there can be system-wide change, involving all or a significant number of medical schools (such as the introduction of laboratory teaching in the basic sciences early in the century).

Minor change has continued throughout the century, and is present today. For example, there is evidence that individual medical schools are making at least minor curricular changes in response to the recommendations of the GPEP Report. A 1989 survey of the 127 accredited U.S. medical schools revealed that since 1984 (the year of the GPEP Report) 95 schools had decreased the number of lecture hours, 104 had introduced or increased independent learning experiences, 106 had introduced or increased small group teaching in the basic sciences, and 90 had introduced or increased the use of outpatient settings for clinical education.[27] While these changes appear to be in the "right direction," the effects of minor changes on the overall education of the student may not be very great. Major change has been less common in recent years, although there have been some well-publicized exceptions such as the curriculum change at Harvard in the mid–1980s.

What does the history of the events surrounding the "Flexner Report" tell current reformers about the possibility of major or system-wide change? First, the environment should support, or at least not inhibit, the change. The environment includes the major professional groups (for example, accrediting agencies and certifying bodies), the government (and associated legislation), the health care delivery system, and the local and regional community of the medical school. While each of these elements may not prove to be important in implementing a given change, all should be considered in the planning process.

Second, the individuals who will be called upon to implement the change should support it, as should medical school leadership. This first requires a perception that problems exist. There was consensus among the leaders of medical education in Flexner's time about the changes needed. These individuals also were in positions within their own medical schools, and within national medical organizations, to ensure administrative and faculty support.

Finally, the change should be logistically feasible, and the necessary resources should be available. For example, introduction of clinical education in the early twentieth century was impossible at some country medical schools without access to hospitals. Similarly, one barrier to the current introduction of small group instruction is the absence of sufficient rooms to divide large classes, and the lack of enough faculty members to serve as group leaders. Logistical problems often can be overcome with some forethought and planning, but will usually be raised as a barrier by those not eager for change. Are there any lessons that can be learned from the early twentieth century that are relevant to current attempts to change medical education? It appears that the specific forces then working to promote change do not support current change efforts. However, the Flexner era tells us that implementing change is a complex process, which requires consideration of many factors besides the educational merits of the innovation. This need for a broad view of change is perhaps the most important lesson we can learn.

Notes

NOTES FOR CHAPTER 1

1. A. Flexner, *Abraham Flexner: An Autobiography* (New York: Simon and Schuster, 1960), p. 79.

2. A. Flexner, *Medical Education in the United States and Canada* (New York: Carnegie Foundation, 1910).

3. A. Bierce, *The Enlarged Devil's Dictionary*, ed. E. J. Hopkins (Garden City, New York: Doubleday and Company, 1967), p. 48.

4. Flexner, *Medical Education, p. 10.*

5. Flexner, *Autobiography*, p. 165.

6. R. P. Hudson, "Patterns of Medical Education in Nineteenth-Century America," Unpublished essay for the M.A. degree, the Johns Hopkins University, 1966. Data derived from H. A. Kelly and W. L. Burrage, *Dictionary of American Medical Biography* (New York: Appleton, 1928). Use of the figures cited from this source requires a *caveat*. The *DAMB* analysis is essentially statistical. This demanded the employment of certain arbitrary definitions and categories which are carefully described in the essay. These should be consulted before any figures or conclusions from the study are used. The analysis contained the reasons individuals were included in the *DAMB*; patterns of premedical, medical, and postgraduate education decade by decade; patterns of age; the influence of economic factors; effects of fathers' occupation, marriage, and educational patterns of the various specialties.

7. T. Bonner, *American Doctors and German Universities: A Chapter in International Intellectual Relations 1870–1914* (Lincoln: University of Nebraska Press, 1963), p. 14.

8. As one example, J. Field pointed out that at least sixteen of the twenty-eight founding members of the American Physiological Society were trained in Germany; *The History of Medical Education*, ed. C. D. O'Malley (Los Angeles: University of California Press, 1970), p. 504.

9. For aspects of this phenomenon see B. J. Stern, *American Medical Practice in the Perspectives of a Century* (New York: The Commonwealth Fund, 1945),

pp. 45–61; H. E. Sigerist, *American Medicine* (New York: W. W. Norton & Company, 1934), pp. 173 ff.; J. S. Haller, Jr., *American Medicine in Transition 1840–1910* (Urbana: University of Illinois Press, 1981), pp. 253–56; and P. Starr, *The Social Transformation of American Medicine,* (New York: Basic Books, 1982), pp. 355–59.

10. A. Flexner, *Daniel Coit Gilman: Creator of the American Type of University* (New York: Harcourt, Brace and Company, 1946), pp. 38–48.

11. M. Kaufman, *American Medical Education: The Formative Years, 1765–1910* (Westport, Connecticut: Greenwood Press, 1976), pp. 150–52.

12. R. H. Shryock, *The Unique Influence of the Johns Hopkins University on American Medicine* (Copenhagen: Munksgaard, 1953).

13. K. M. Ludmerer, *Learning to Heal: The Development of American Medical Education* (New York: Basic Books, 1985), pp. 40–46, 108–13.

14. R. H. Fitz, "The Legislative Control of Medical Practice," *Medical Communications of the Massachusetts Medical Society,* 16 (1894): 306–07. For a consideration of the sectarian movement in general, see J. F. Kett, *The Formation of the American Medical Profession: The Role of Institutions, 1780–1860* (New Haven: Yale University Press, 1968) and W. G. Rothstein, *American Physicians in the Nineteenth Century: From Sects to Science* (Baltimore: Johns Hopkins University Press, 1972).

15. Fitz, "Legislative Control," pp. 282 ff.

16. The history of therapy has been neglected in the past, but the situation is improving. See A. Berman, "The Heroic Approach in 19th-Century Therapeutics," in *Sickness and Health in America: Readings in the History of Medicine and Public Health,* ed. J. W. Leavitt and R. L. Numbers (Madison: University of Wisconsin Press, 1978), pp. 77–86; C. E. Rosenberg, "The Therapeutic Revolution: Medicine, Meaning, and Social Change in 19th-Century America," in *Sickness and Health,* 2nd ed. 1985, pp. 39–52, and J. H. Warner, *The Therapeutic Perspective: Medical Practice, Knowledge, and Identity in America, 1820–1885* (Cambridge: Harvard University Press, 1986).

17. R. H. Shryock, *The Development of Modern Medicine* (Madison: University of Wisconsin Press, 1979), pp. 258–62.

18. N. S. Davis, *History of the American Medical Association* (Philadelphia: Lippincott, Grambo and Co., 1855), pp. 34–39, 115–18. See also J. G. Burrow, *Organized Medicine in the Progressive Era: The Move Toward Monopoly* (Baltimore: Johns Hopkins University Press, 1977).

19. D. F. Smiley, "History of the Association of American Medical Colleges, 1896–1956," *Journal of Medical Education* 32 (1957): 512–25.

20. C. B. Chapman, "*The Flexner Report* by Abraham Flexner," *Daedalus* 103 (Winter 1973): 105–17.

21. G. H. Brieger, "The Flexner Report: Revised or Revisited?" *Medical Heritage* 1 (1985): 25.

22. Flexner, *Medical Education,* p. 151.

23. "Medical Education in the United States: Annual Presentation of Educational Data for 1930 by the Council on Medical Education and Hospitals," *JAMA* 95 (1930): 504.

24. Ibid., p. 504.

25. *Historical Statistics of the United States: Colonial Times to 1957* (Washington, D.C.: U. S. Government Printing Office, 1961), p. 34.

26. *Contributions to the History of Medical Education and Medical Institutions in the United States of America 1776–1876* (Washington, D.C.: Government Printing Office, 1877), pp. 41–42.

27. Stern, *American Medical Practice*, p. 63.

28. Flexner, *Medical Education*, p. 14.

29. *Excerpts from the AMA Physician Masterfile*, November, 1984, p. 4; and *The World Almanac and Book of Facts* (New York: Newspaper Enterprise Association, 1985), p. 246.

30. Flexner, *Medical Education*, pp. 28–51. The quote is on p. 30.

31. Ibid., pp. 23–27.

32. Flexner, *Medical Education: A Comparative Study*, (New York: Macmillan Company, 1925), p. 79.

33. Ibid., p. 86.

34. *Physicians for the Twenty-First Century* (Washington, D.C.: Association of American Medical Colleges, 1984).

35. Flexner, *Medical Education*, p. 56.

36. J. Burnham, "American Medicine's Golden Age: What Happened to It?" *Science* 215 (1982): 1474–79.

37. Flexner, *Medical Education*, p. 56.

38. Ibid., pp. 56–57.

39. R. Hofstadter and C. D. Hardy, *The Development and Scope of Higher Education in the United States* (New York: Columbia University Press, 1952), p. 64. The figures given are 198 in 1871; 2,382 in 1890 and 9,370 in 1910.

40. Flexner, *Medical Education*, p. 72.

41. Ibid., pp. 91–93.

42. Ibid., pp. 99–100.

43. Ludmerer, *Learning to Heal*, pp. 156–60.

44. Ibid., pp. 219–33.

45. G. W. Corner, *Two Centuries of Medicine: A History of the School of Medicine, University of Pennsylvania* (Philadelphia: J. B. Lippincott Company, 1965), p. 24.

46. New York was in the vanguard in returning to control of medical practice. For the complexities of this seesaw battle, see J. B. Bardo, "A History of the Legal Regulation of Medical Practice in New York State," *Bulletin of the New York Academy of Medicine* 43 (1967): 923–40. See also R. H. Shryock, *Medical Licensing in America, 1650–1965* (Baltimore: Johns Hopkins University Press, 1967) and R. C. Derbyshire, *Medical Licensure and Disciplines in the United States* (Baltimore: Johns Hopkins University Press, 1969).

47. Fitz, "Legislative Control," pp. 294, 313.

48. Flexner, *Medical Education*, p. 167.

49. L. S. King, "The Flexner Report of 1910," *JAMA* 251 (1984): 1079–86. For an analysis that is unfortunately too often overlooked in this regard, see S. Jarcho, "Medical Education in the United States, 1910–1956," *Journal of the Mt. Sinai Hospital* 26 (1959): 339–85. Also, H. D. Banta, "Abraham Flexner—A Reappraisal," *Social Science and Medicine* 5 (1971): 655–61; D. M. Fox, "Abraham Flexner's Unpublished Report: Foundations and Medical Education, 1909–1928," *Bulletin History of Medicine* 54 (1980): 475–96; and H. S. Berliner, "A Larger Perspective on the Flexner Report," *International Journal of the Health Sciences* 5 (1975): 573–92.

50. Ludmerer, *Learning to Heal,* p. 50.

51. R. P. Hudson, "Abraham Flexner in Perspective: American Medical Education 1865–1910," *Bulletin of the History of Medicine,* 46 (1972): 545.

52. Chapman, *"The Flexner Report," passim,* esp. p. 111.

53. Berliner, "A Larger Perspective," pp. 587–90.

54. Ludmerer, *Learning to Heal,* pp. 200–06.

55. Berliner, "A Larger Perspective," *passim,* and *A System of Scientific Medicine: Philanthropic Foundations in the Flexner Era* (New York: Tavistock Publications, 1985); and E. R. Brown, *Rockefeller Medicine Men: Medicine and Capitalism in America* (Berkeley: University of California Press, 1979).

56. Berliner, "A Larger Perspective," and *Scientific Medicine, passim.*

57. Berliner, *Scientific Medicine,* p. 78.

58. D. M. Fox, "Recent Marxist Interpretations of the History of Medicine in the United States," *Clio Medica* 16 (1982): 225. Starr, *The Social Transformation of American Medicine,* rejects the Marxist argument as well, pp. 16–17 and 462, n. 103.

59. Ludmerer, *Learning to Heal,* pp. 84–87, 101, 141.

60. H. L. Mencken, quoted in J. M. Cohen and M. J. Cohen, *The Penguin Dictionary of Modern Quotations,* 2nd ed., (New York: Penguin Books, 1980), p. 229.

61. Berliner, *Scientific Medicine,* p. 113.

62. Flexner, *Medical Education,* p. 143.

63. Brieger, "The Flexner Report."

64. P. Ward, "The Other Abraham: Flexner in Illinois," *Caduceus: A Quarterly for the Health Sciences* 2 (Spring, 1986): 1–55.

65. D. B. Munger, "Robert Brookings and the Flexner Report: A Case Study of the Reorganization of Medical Education," *Journal of the History of Medicine and Allied Sciences* 23 (1968): 356–71. See also Flexner, *Autobiography,* pp. 81–83.

66. See, for example, Berliner, *Scientific Medicine,* p. 108.

67. Flexner, *Autobiography,* p. 45.

68. Ibid., pp. 232–49.

69. Flexner, *Medical Education: A Comparative Study,* pp. 137–38.

70. Brieger, "The Flexner Report," p. 29.

71. Ludmerer, *Learning to Heal,* p. 7.

NOTES FOR CHAPTER 2

1. G. Berry, "Medical Education in Transition," *Journal of Medical Education* 28 (1953): 17.

2. N. S. Davis, *Contributions to the History of Medical Education and Medical Institutions in the United States of America, 1776–1876* (Washington, D.C.: Government Printing Office, 1877), p. 45; F. C. Waite, "Advent of the Graded Curriculum in American Medical Colleges," *Journal of the Association of American Medical Colleges* 25 (1950): 315–22.

3. A. Flexner, *Medical Education in the United States and Canada* (New York City: Carnegie Foundation for the Advancement of Teaching, 1910), pp. 24–25, 61.

4. *AAMC Curriculum Directory 1989–1990* (Washington, D.C.: Association of American Medical Colleges, 1989).

5. Flexner, *Medical Education,* pp. 53–56.

6. Ibid., pp. 60–61.

7. Ibid., pp. 56–57.

8. Ibid., pp. 57–59.

9. Ibid., p. 76.

10. Ibid., p. 61.

11. *A Model Medical Curriculum* (Chicago: Council on Medical Education, 1909), pp. 14–16, 44–45; Flexner, *Medical Education,* pp. 61–68.

12. Flexner, *Medical Education,* p. 90.

13. H. A. Christian, "The Concentration Plan of Teaching Medicine," *Proceedings of the Association of American Medical Colleges* 20 (1910): 31–35, 37–39.

14. Flexner, *Medical Education,* p. 69.

15. Ibid., pp. 29, 74–89.

16. Ibid., p. 88.

17. "Work for a Standard Curriculum in Medical Education," *AMA Bulletin* 5 (1909): 16–24; "AAMC Report of the Committee on Curriculum," *JAMA* 54 (1910): 1227–28.

18. W. Welch, "The Medical Curriculum," *Proceedings of the Association of American Medical Colleges Twentieth Annual Meeting* (1910): 62.

19. A. D. Bevan, "The Modern School of Medicine," *AMA Bulletin* 7 (1912): 145.

20. W. H. Howell, "The Medical School as Part of the University," in *Medical Research and Education,* vol. 2, ed. J.M. Cattell (New York: The Science Press, 1913), p. 201.

21. In 1925, there were 80 medical schools in the U.S., compared to 131 in 1910 and 160 in 1900. Of the schools in 1925, 9 offered only the first 2 years of the curriculum and 71 had 4-year programs. Commission on Medical Education, *Final Report* (New York: Office of the Director of the Study, 1932), Table 104.

22. *Final Report,* pp. 181–82.

23. F. Zapffe, "The Curriculum," *Proceedings of the Association of American Medical Colleges* 35 (1925): 142–43.

24. *Final Report,* p. 174; Zapffe, "The Curriculum," pp. 142–43.

25. A. Flexner, *Medical Education: A Comparative Study* (New York: The Macmillan Company, 1925), p. 142.

26. *Final Report,* p. 181; H. Cabot, "Report on Curriculum," *Proceedings of the Association of American Medical Colleges* 33 (1923): 157.

27. A. Mathews, "Twenty Years of Growth and Development in Biochemistry," *AMA Papers and Discussion/Congress on Medical Education and Licensure* (1925): 12; C. Guthrie, "Twenty Years of Progress in Physiology and Pharmacology," *AMA Papers and Discussion/Congress on Medical Education and Licensure* (1925): 14.

28. *Final Report,* p. 174.

29. *Final Report,* p. 174; A. D. Bevan, "Needed Developments in Medical Education," *AMA Bulletin* 14 (1920): 6.

30. *Choice of a Medical School* (Chicago: American Medical Association, 1925), pp. 9–10.

31. J. Erlanger et al., "An Investigation of Conditions in the Departments of the Preclinical Sciences," *JAMA* 74 (1920): 1117–20; C. Jackson, "Progress in Anatomy Since 1900," *AMA Papers and Discussion/Congress on Medical Education and Licensure* (1925): 7–8.

32. H. Cabot, "Report of the Committee on Curriculum of the Association of American Medical Colleges," *Proceedings of the Thirty-Second Annual AAMC Meeting* (1922): 78; *Final Report*, Table 112.

33. "Council on Medical Education and Hospitals of the AMA," *Journal of the Association of American Medical Colleges* 10 (1935): 191–92.

34. In 1940 there were 67 4-year medical schools and 10 that had only a 2-year (basic science) program. "Medical Education in the United States and Canada," *JAMA* 115 (1940): 685–708; H. G. Weiskotten et al., *Medical Education in the United States, 1934–1939* (Chicago: American Medical Association, 1940), pp. 127, 135; R. L. Wilbur, "Survey of Medical Education," *Journal of the Association of American Medical Colleges* 9 (1934): 180–81.

35. *Medical Education in the U.S.*, pp. 85, 122–23, 133, 140, 149, 157, 163.

36. Ibid., pp. 85, 137.

37. L. Clements, "Objectives in Teaching Anatomy," *Journal of the Association of American Medical Colleges* 14 (1939): 170–74.

38. *Medical Education in the U.S.*, pp. 82, 121, 130, 138, 148, 156, 161; F. Zapffe, "Number of Physicians and Others Connected with the Faculties of the Medical Schools of the United States and Canada," *Journal of the Association of American Medical Colleges* 11 (1936): 350–56.

39. *Medical Education in the U.S.*, pp. 80–81.

40. In 1955 there were 75 4-year medical schools and 6 2-year schools. E. Turner, W. Wiggins, and A. Tipner, "Medical Education in the United States and Canada," *JAMA* 159 (1955): 565.

41. "Medical Education in the United States and Canada," *JAMA* 153 (1953): 106–08; see, *The Teaching of Physiology, Biochemistry and Pharmacology: Report of the First Teaching Institute* (Chicago: Association of American Medical Colleges, 1954); *The Teaching of Pathology, Microbiology, Immunology and Genetics: Report of the Second Teaching Institute* (Chicago: Association of American Medical Colleges, 1955); *The Teaching of Anatomy and Anthropology in Medical Education: Report of the Third Teaching Institute* (Chicago: Association of American Medical Colleges, 1956).

42. J. Deitrick and R. Berson, *Medical Schools in the United States at Mid-Century* (Evanston, Illinois: Association of American Medical Colleges, 1960), pp. 259–60; E. Turner et al., "Medical Education in the United States and Canada," *JAMA* 161 (1956): 1646–48; M. Senn and F. Stricker, *An Appraisal of Undergraduate Medical Education in the United States with Reference to the Teaching of Medical Psychology* (Geneva: World Health Organization, 1953).

43. M. Bussigel, B. Barzansky and G. Grenholm, *Innovation Processes in Medical Education* (New York, Praeger Publishing Company, 1988), pp. 45–56.

44. In 1950, there were a total of 2,614 faculty members with the rank of instructor or above in the basic science departments and about 14,000 first- and second-year medical students. J. Hinsey, "Maintenance of a Continuing Supply of New Faculty Members," in *Medical Education Today*, ed. D. Smiley (Chicago: Association of American Medical Colleges, 1953), pp. 6–21.

45. "Undergraduate Medical Education," *JAMA* 218 (1971): 1204, 1217.

46. V. Lippard, "Trends in the Medical Curriculum," in *The Changing Medical Curriculum,* ed. V. Lippard and E. Purcell (New York: Josiah Macy Jr. Foundation, 1972), pp. 13–14; G. DeMuth and J. Gronvall, "The Questionnaire and its Analysis," *Journal of Medical Education* 45 (no. 11, part 2, 1970): 17–18; M. Visscher, "The Decline in Emphasis on Basic Medical Sciences in Medical School Curricula," *The Physiologist* 16 (1973): 52.

47. *AAMC Curriculum Directory* 1972/1973 (Washington, D.C.: Association of American Medical Colleges, 1972).

48. *AAMC Curriculum Directory* 1974/1975 (Washington, D.C.: Association of American Medical Colleges, 1974).

49. In 1970, there were 8,053 full-time faculty members with the rank of instructor and above in basic science departments (as compared to 2,614 in 1955). The average number of full-time faculty ranged from 17 in pathology departments to 9 in pharmacology and microbiology departments. In 1971–72, 33 percent of anatomy department heads, 17 percent of biochemistry department heads, 45 percent of physiology department heads, 43 percent of microbiology department heads, 99 percent of pathology department heads, and 63 percent of pharmacology department heads were physicians. "Undergraduate Medical Education," *Journal of the Association of American Medical Colleges* 218 (1971): 1214; Datagram: Medical School Staffing Patterns," *Journal of Medical Education* 45 (1970): 681; *Directory of American Medical Education* (Washington, D.C.: Association of American Medical Colleges), 1971.

50. Council on Medical Education, *Future Directions for Medical Education* (Chicago: American Medical Association, 1982); "Physicians for the Twenty-First Century," *Journal of Medical Education* 54 (no. 11, part 2, 1984).

51. *AAMC Curriculum Directory* 1984/1985 (Washington, D.C.: Association of American Medical Colleges, 1984); H. Jonas, S. Etzel, and B. Barzansky, "Undergraduate Medical Education," *JAMA* 262 (1989): 1018.

52. *AAMC Curriculum Directories* for 1983/1984, 1986/1987, and 1989/1990.

53. In 1985, there were 13,783 full-time faculty members with the rank of instructor and above in basic science departments. The average number of faculty members per department ranged from 13 in pharmacology departments to 31 in pathology departments. Crowley, et al., "Undergraduate Medical Education," p. 1565; *Directory of American Medical Education 1983/1984,* (Washington, D.C.: Association of American Medical Colleges, 1983).

54. Bussigel, et al., *Innovation Processes in Medical Education,* pp. 126–29.

NOTES FOR CHAPTER 3

1. A. Flexner, *Medical Education in the United States and Canada* (New York: Carnegie Foundation, 1910), p. 346.

2. A. Flexner, *I Remember* (New York: Simon and Schuster, 1940), p. 285.

3. At least twenty-three schools had deans who were not clinicians; pathologists and physiologists predominated.

4. Letter of W. Osler to W. S. Thayer, August 6, 1904. Quoted in H. Cushing, *The Life of Osler,* vol. 1 (Oxford: Oxford University Press, 1925) pp. 650–51.

5. For a graphic illustration of these changes see E. C. Atwater, "A Modest

but Good Institution . . . and Besides there is Mr. Eastman," in *To Each His Farthest Star—University of Rochester Medical Center 1925–1975*. (Rochester, New York: Rochester University Press, 1975), p. 29.

6. Quoted in F. R. Sabin, *Franklin Paine Mall, The Story of a Mind* (Baltimore: Johns Hopkins University Press, 1934), p. 270.

7. Letter of Osler to Pres. Remsen (of Johns Hopkins) on the subject of whole-time clinical professors. Quoted in A. M. Chesney, *The Johns Hopkins Hospital and the Johns Hopkins University School of Medicine, A Chronicle*, vol. 3 (Baltimore: Johns Hopkins University Press, 1963), pp. 177–83.

8. E. C. Atwater, "Family Medicine, Boston Style," *Harvard Medical Alumni Bulletin* 57 (1983): 31–36.

9. E. C. Atwater, "Touching the Patient: The Teaching of Internal Medicine in America," in *Sickness and Health in America, Readings in the History of Medicine and Public Health*," 2 ed., ed. J. W. Leavitt and R. L. Numbers (Madison: University of Wisconsin Press, 1985), pp. 129–47.

10. D. J. DeSolla Price, *Little Science, Big Science* (New York: Columbia University Press, 1963).

11. The story of the development of clinical research in hospitals is well documented in J. C. Aub and R. K. Hapgood, *Pioneer in Modern Medicine, David Linn Edsall of Harvard* (Boston: Harvard Medical Alumni Association 1970); A. M. Harvey, *Science at the Bedside, Clinical Research in American Medicine 1905–1954* (Baltimore and London: Johns Hopkins University Press, 1981); and J. H. Means, *Ward 4, the Mallinckrodt Research Ward of the Massachusetts General Hospital* (Cambridge: Harvard University Press 1958).

12. Though Walter B. Cannon is generally credited with proposing the use of the case method of teaching clinical medicine, the idea was apparently coming into use in several places at the turn of the century. See E. C. Atwater, "Making Fewer Mistakes," *Bulletin of the History of Medicine* 57 (1983): 178.

13. L. A. Kohn, "The Place of the Practitioner in the Teaching of Medicine," *American Practitioner and Digest of Treatment* 4 (1953): 552–54.

14. Atwater, "Touching the Patient," p. 142.

15. See, for example, R. H. Ebert and E. Ginzberg, "The Reform of Medical Education," *Health Affairs* 7 (Supplement 1988): 17, 32.

16. Atwater, "Making Fewer Mistakes," pp. 165–87.

17. J. A. Curran, "Internships and Residencies: Historical Backgrounds and Current Trends," *Journal of Medical Education* 34 (1959): 879.

18. B. N. Carter. "Fruition of Halsted's Concept of Surgical Training," *Surgery* 32 (1952): 518–27.

19. Curran, "Internships and Residencies," p. 879.

20. See, for example, *1989–1990 Directory of Graduate Medical Education Programs* (Chicago: ACGME, 1989).

21. Barbara W. Tuchman, *The Guns of August* (New York: Bantam, 1976) pp. 15–18; Henry Adams, *Mont-Saint-Michel and Chartres* (Boston: Houghton Mifflin Company, 1913); Upton Sinclair, *The Jungle* (New York: Grosset and Dunlap, 1906).

22. The teacher is not included here since medicine does not recognize the teacher per se, no matter how excellent, but only the investigator or practitioner who teaches.

NOTES FOR CHAPTER 4

1. K. Ludmerer, *Learning to Heal: The Development of American Medical Education* (New York: Basic Books, Inc., 1985), p. 248.

2. For work by other scholars, see R. Shryock, *Medical Licensing in America, 1650–1965* (Baltimore: Johns Hopkins University Press, 1967), p. 377; B. Ehrenreich and D. English, "Witches, Midwives and Nurses," *Monthly Review* 25 (October 1973): 36–37; Ehrenreich and English, *For Her Own Good; 150 Years of Experts' Advice to Women* (New York: Anchor Press/Doubleday, 1978), p. 79; J. Leeson and J. Gray, *Women and Medicine* (London: Tavistock Publications, 1987), p. 28; J. B. Litoff, *American Midwives: 1860 to the Present* (Westport, Connecticut: Greenwood Press, 1978), p. 49; G. Markowitz and D. Rosner, "Doctors in Crisis: Medical Education and Medical Reform During the Progressive Era, 1895–1915," in *Health Care in America: Essays in Social History,* ed. S. Reverby and D. Rosner (Philadelphia: Temple University Press, 1979), p. 196. The error that the "Flexner Report" caused women's demise in medicine has also been repeated by other authors. P. Starr, *The Social Transformation of American Medicine* (New York: Basic Books, 1982) is an exception to this generalization.

3. M. R. Walsh, *Doctors Wanted: No Women Need Apply* (New Haven: Yale University Press, 1977), pp. 239–40.

4. Ibid., p. xvii.

5. W. Rothstein, *American Medical Schools and the Practice of Medicine* (New York: Oxford University Press, 1987), pp. 115, 290.

6. Faye Crosby, unpublished paper delivered at the New England Social Psychological Association Meeting, Yale University, New Haven, Connecticut Sept. 26, 1987. This growing scholarly literature includes D. Rhode, "The Evolution of Sex Discrimination Law," unpublished Manuscript; *Sex-based Discrimination: Text, Cases and Materials,* ed. Herma Kay (St. Paul, Minnesota: West Publishing Company, 1981); *1986 Supplement to Text, Cases and Materials on Sex-Based Discrimination,* ed. Herma Kay, 2d ed. (St. Paul, Minnesota: West Publishing Company, 1986); A. Sachs and J. Wilson, *Sexism and the Law: A Study of Male Beliefs and Legal Bias in Britain and the United States* (New York: The Free Press, 1978); N. Benokraitis and J. Feagin, *Modern Sexism: Blatant, Subtle and Covert Discrimination* (Englewood Cliffs, New Jersey: Prentice-Hall, 1986). Other excellent studies are appearing which integrate the study of prejudice against women with patterns of ethnic and religious discrimination. See, for example, D. Oren, *Joining the Club: A History of Jews and Yale* (New Haven, Connecticut: Yale University Press, 1985).

7. Walsh, *Doctors Wanted,* pp. 8–9. There is a dispute about whether Walter Channing wrote this document or whether it was written by John Ware, another obstetrician in Boston. For the argument that the author is John Ware, see E. Manzer, "Woman's Doctors: The Development of Obstetrics and Gynecology in Boston, 1860–1930," unpublished doctoral dissertation, Indiana University, Bloomington, Indiana 1979, pp. 15–20. I am not persuaded by the argument crediting Ware. Since both men were Boston obstetricians, the actual identity of the author is not relevant to the point being made.

8. Walsh, *Doctors Wanted,* pp. 110–11.

9. A. Vietor, pp. 404–05, cited in *Send Us a Lady Physician: Women Doctors in America, 1835–1920,* ed. R. J. Abraham (New York: W. W. Norton and Company, 1985), p. 102.

10. Walsh, *Doctors Wanted,* pp. 14–15.

11. Ibid., pp. 1, 14, 22–27.

12. B. Riznik, "Medicine in New England 1790–1840," unpublished manuscript, Countway Medical Library of Harvard University, Cambridge, Massachusetts, p. 117; Walsh, *Doctors Wanted,* Chapter 1. My thesis on women doctors has been confirmed by other scholars. See, for example R. Morantz-Sanchez, *Sympathy and Science: Women Physicians in American Medicine* (New York: Oxford University Press, 1985) and G. Moldow, *Women Doctors in Gilded-Age Washington: Race, Gender and Professionalization* (Champaign, Illinois: University of Illinois Press, 1987). Both authors provide detailed discussions of the discrimination against women that pervaded medical education.

13. Walsh, *Doctors Wanted,* pp. 14–15.

14. Walsh, *Doctors Wanted,* pp. 238–39.

15. Walsh, *Doctors Wanted,* chapter 6. *Records of the Commissioner of Education* includes statistics on all the medical schools for this historical period with gender distinctions for both enrolled students and graduates.

16. "General Circular (for Women's Committee for Johns Hopkins Medical School)," separate editions published in the spring and fall of 1890, Sophie Smith Collection, Smith College, Northampton, Massachusetts; Johns Hopkins University Circular, Catalogue and Announcement for 1910–1911 of Medical Department, 1910, pp. 174–80; Alan Chesney, *The Johns Hopkins University School of Medicine,* vol. 1 and 2, (Baltimore: Johns Hopkins University Press, 1943 and 1958); *Retrospect of Twenty Years of Johns Hopkins Medical School, 1876–1896,* (Baltimore: Johns Hopkins University Press, 1896), p. 38.

17. *Women's Medical Journal* 6 (1899): 249; E. Blackwell, "The New York Infirmary and College," *Transactions of the Woman's Medical College of Pennsylvania* (1900): 80.

18. Dec. 26, 1917, Joseph Erlanger Manuscripts, Washington University Medical School, St. Louis; cited in Morantz-Sanchez, *Sympathy and Science,* pp. 253–54.

19. *Women's Medical Journal* 11 (1901): 13; *Transactions of the Woman's Medical College of Pennsylvania* (1900): 19; *Transactions of the Woman's Medical College of Pennsylvania (1912): 78; Walsh, Doctors Wanted,* p. 263.

20. Both Ludmerer, in *Learning to Heal,* and Rothstein, in *American Medical Schools,* provide information on medical school faculty members, yet there still is no definitive study on the topic. Morantz-Sanchez, *Sympathy and Science,* provides some glimpses of what it may have been like for women faculty, but she deals primarily with women who taught at women's medical schools. Even for the contemporary period, we have only limited research on teaching faculty in medical schools.

21. *Transactions of the Woman's Medical College of Pennsylvania* (1901): 14; Walsh, *Doctors Wanted,* p. 279.

22. *Transactions of the Women's Medical College of Pennsylvania* (1912): 78, cited in Walsh, *Doctors Wanted,* p. 263.

23. From Mendenhall Manuscript Autobiography in Sophie Smith Collection,

Smith College. The Mosher and Mendenhall cases are cited in Morantz-Sanchez, *Sympathy and Science,* p. 100.

24. M. Duberman, *The Uncompleted Past* (New York: Random House 1969), p. 8; T. Miller, "Male Attitudes Toward Women's Rights as a Function of Their Level of Self-Esteem," paper read at the 80th annual convention of the American Psychological Association, Division 9 Symposium: Who Discriminates Against Women?, Honolulu, Hawaii, September 1972.

25. These men are discussed more fully in Walsh, *Doctors Wanted,* pp. 147–77, where extensive references to their writings also appear.

26. A. Flexner, *Medical Education in the United States and Canada* (New York: Carnegie Foundation, 1910), pp. 178–79. Overall, Ludmerer's background account of the "Flexner Report" in *Learning to Heal* is an excellent one (pp. 166–90). Although I disagree with him about the impact of the "Flexner Report" on women, he provides a very comprehensive discussion of other issues. For additional documentation on sex discrimination, see R. Morantz-Sanchez, *Sympathy and Science* and G. Moldow, *Women Doctors in Gilded-Age Washington.*

27. See *JAMA* 57 (1911).

28. S. Baserga, "The Early Years of Coeducation at the Yale University School of Medicine," *The Yale Journal of Biology and Medicine* 53 (1989): 184–85; Walsh, *Doctors Wanted,* pp. 176–77.

29. L. Arey, *Northwestern University Medical School 1859–1959: A Pioneer in Educational Reform* (Chicago: Northwestern University Press, 1959) pp. 120–22, 214, 441–42, cited in Walsh, *Doctors Wanted,* p. 205.

30. *AMA Directory for 1921*; Walsh, *Doctors Wanted,* p. 224.

31. B. Van Hoosen, "Opportunities for Women Medical Interns," *Women's Medical Journal* 33 (1926): 102–05, 194–96.

32. Jacqueline Seaver, "Women Doctors in Spite of Everything," *The New York Times Magazine* 31 (March 31, 1961): 67.

33. L. Haignere, "Admission of Women to Medical Schools: A Study of Organizational Response to Social Movement and Public Policy Pressures," unpublished doctoral dissertation, University of Connecticut, Storrs, Connecticut, p. 155.

34. The poster is described in *Project on the Status of and Education of Women,* University of Hawaii, unpublished pp. 2–3.

35. Stanford recruitment brochure undated (about 1973), is located in the Office of Career Services, Harvard University.

36. "Obstacles to Equal Education at Harvard Medical School Resulting from Sex Discrimination" (1974), published by Harvard University and available from the Harvard Medical School Joint Committee on the Status of Women.

37. Estelle Ramey's letter of Aug. 1, 1972 was directed to the membership of the Association of Women in Science; R. F. Becker, J. W. Wilson and J. A. Gehweiler, *The Anatomical Basis of Medical Practice* (Baltimore: Williams and Wilkins, 1971), pp. vii, 128.

38. Walsh, *Doctors Wanted,* p. 111.

39. A. Schuller et al., "Suicide Among United States Women Physicians," *American Journal of Psychiatry* 136 (1979): 694–96.

40. Letters (December 1979), *American Journal of Psychiatry* 161 (1979): 695.

41. Schuller et al., "Suicide Among United States Women Physicians," pp. 694–96.

42. A. Scheneman, J. Pickelman and R. Freeark, "Age, Gender, Lateral Dominance, and the Prediction of Operative Skill Among General Surgery Residents," *Surgery* 98 (1985): 506–13.

43. H. Polk, "Discussion," *Surgery* 98 (1985): 514.

44. G. Baillie, "Should Professional Women Marry," *Women's Medical Journal* 2 (February 1894): 33–35, cited by Morantz-Sanchez, *Sympathy and Science*, p. 130.

45. M. Sayers et al., "Pregnancy During Residency," *New England Journal of Medicine* 314 (1986): 3.

46. "Stanford Physician Quits After Criticizing Pregnancy," *Chronicle of Higher Education* 25 (Jan. 18, 1984): 3.

47. M. Sayers, "Mothers and Fathers of Invention," *Harvard Medical Alumni Bulletin* 60 (Spring 1986): 20–21.

48. D. Kirp, M. Yudof and M. Franks, *Gender Justice* (Chicago: University of Chicago Press, 1986), p. 41.

NOTES FOR CHAPTER 5

1. Little has been written on the early history of black medical schools (through 1920). Some information is available in: H. M. Morais, *The History of the Negro in Medicine* (New York: Publishers Company, Inc., 1967), pp. 39–48, 59–88; W. M. Cobb, *Progress and Portents for the Negro in Medicine* (New York: NAACP, 1948); C. V. Roman, *Meharry Medical College: A History* (Nashville: Sunday School Publishing Board of the National Baptist Convention, 1934); J. Summerville, *Educating Black Doctors: A History of Meharry Medical College* (University, Alabama: University of Alabama Press, 1983); D. C. Hine, "The Pursuit of Professional Equality: Meharry Medical College, 1921–1938, A Case Study," in *New Perspectives on Black Educational History*, ed. V. P. Franklin and J. D. Anderson (Boston: G. K. Hall, 1978), pp. 173–92; L. A. Falk and H. A. Quaynor-Malm, "Early Afro-American Medical Education in the United States: The Origins of Meharry Medical College in the Nineteenth Century," in *Proceedings of the XXIII Congress of the History of Medicine* (London, 1972), pp. 346–56; *Howard University Medical Department, Washington, D.C.: A Historical, Biographical and Statistical Souvenir*, comp. and ed. D. S. Lamb (Washington, D.C.: R. Beresford, 1900); W. Dyson, *Founding the School of Medicine of Howard University, 1868–1873*, (Howard University Studies in History, no. 10 (Washington, D.C., 1929); Dyson, *Howard University, The Capstone of Negro Education, A History: 1867–1940* (Washington, D.C.: Howard University Graduate School, 1941), pp. 44–49, 239–86; Todd L. Savitt, "The Education of Black Physicians at Shaw University, 1882–1918," in *Black Americans in North Carolina and the South*, ed. J. J. Crow and F. J. Hatley (Chapel Hill, N.C.: University of North Carolina Press, 1984), pp. 160–88; D. C. Hine, "The Anatomy of Failure: Medical Education Reform and the Leonard Medical School of Shaw University, 1882–1920," *Journal of Negro Education* 54 (1985): 512–25; Savitt, "Lincoln University Medical Department—A Forgotten 19th-Century Black Medical School," *Journal of the History of Medicine and Allied Sciences* 40 (1985): 42–65; M. V. Lynk, *Sixty Years of Medicine or The Life and Time*

of *Dr. Miles V. Lynk, An Autobiography* (Memphis: The Twentieth Century Press, 1951).

2. On the medical education reform era, see K. M. Ludmerer, *Learning to Heal: The Development of American Medical Education* (New York: Basic Books, 1985); R. P. Hudson, "Abraham Flexner in Perspective: American Medical Education, 1865–1910," *Bulletin of the History of Medicine* 56 (1972): 545–61; M. Kaufman, *American Medical Education: The Formative Years, 1765–1910* (Westport, Conn.: Greenwood Press, 1976).

3. C. F. Meserve to W. Buttrick, May 25, 1907, GEB Papers, Box 103, Folder 929, Rockefeller Archive Center (hereafter cited as RAC), Tarrytown, New York.

4. For an example of the way these problems affected one black medical school, see Savitt, "Education of Black Physicians."

5. See for example, Hudson, "Abraham Flexner in Perspective," p. 545.

6. *JAMA* 48 (1907): 1702.

7. *JAMA* 46 (1906): 1854–56, 47 (1906): 595.

8. *JAMA* 48 (1907): 1704–05.

9. See, for example, *JAMA* 47 (1906): 597–98; 48 (1907): 1702, 1706.

10. Catalogues of the various black medical schools give details of improvements each year though, as Flexner (*Medical Education in the United States and Canada*) stated in his report on Knoxville Medical College (p. 304), the information was not always accurate. See also ABHMS Trustees Minutes, May 6, 1904, in Minutebook, 1902–1917, Shaw University Archives, Raleigh, N.C.

11. *JAMA* 48 (1907): 1603–04.

12. *JAMA* 48 (1907): 1702–03; 50 (1908): 1544.

13. *JAMA* 48 (1907): 1706.

14. See for example, ibid. Ludmerer, *Learning to Heal*, pp. 80–87, shows how many white schools of the time voluntarily made advances in their education program despite the cost. Black schools for the most part could not do this, though they did implement what reforms they felt feasible, as they did not have the financial strength to survive the several lean years until enrollments grew again.

15. *JAMA* 48 (1907): 1702.

16. For more on LMS problems, see Savitt, "Education of Black Physicians."

17. See faculty lists and other information in catalogues of these schools.

18. *JAMA* 48 (1907): 1702.

19. *JAMA* 48 (1907): 1702; 63 (1914): 668.

20. C. F. Meserve to W. Buttrick, May 25, 1907, GEB Papers, Box 103, Folder 929, RAC.

21. No records of this school have been located. See H. J. Abrahams, *The Extinct Medical Schools of Baltimore, Maryland* (Baltimore: Maryland Historical Society, 1969), pp. 324–25. Thanks to Ms. D. Wolverton, librarian at the Medical and Chirurgical Faculty of the State of Maryland, Baltimore, for her help in locating information on this school.

22. See catalogues of State University, LNMC, and correspondence and reports on State University in GEB Papers, Box 74, Folder 648, RAC. Information on Simmons College may be found in L. H. Williams, *Black Higher Education in Kentucky, 1879–1930: The History of Simmons University* (Lewiston/Queenston, Kentucky: Edwin Mellen Press, 1986).

23. No catalogues of Chattanooga National Medical College have been located. Some information may be found in Chattanooga city directories of the time and the medical college listings at the start of each edition of the *American Medical Directory* beginning in 1906.

24. Untitled Report, June 1, 1908, Abraham Flexner Papers, Box 21, "Professional Education—Misc.," Library of Congress, Washington, D.C.

25. *JAMA* 50 (1908): 1543–46.

26. A. Flexner, *Medical Education in the United States and Canada* (New York: Carnegie Foundation, 1910).

27. For an example of the manner in which a white medical journal ignored a black medical school, see issues of the *North Carolina Medical Journal* during the late nineteenth century. It mentions LMS only incidentally.

28. Flexner, *Medical Educatio*, p. 280.

29. Ibid., p. 305.

30. Ibid., pp. 303–04.

31. Ibid., p. 280.

32. Ibid., p. 233.

33. Ibid., p. 304.

34. Ibid., p. 309.

35. Ibid., p. 303.

36. Ibid., p. 304.

37. Ibid., p. 280.

38. Ibid., p. 232.

39. Ibid., p. 305.

40. Ibid., pp. 180–81.

41. Ibid., p. 180.

42. Ibid., p. 181.

43. New Orleans University *Catalogue,* 1911/1912, p. 24.

44. *JAMA* 59 (1912): 642.

45. *Journal of the National Medical Association* 1 (1909): 257–58; 2 (1910): 23–29.

46. For information on the school, see Lynk, *Sixty Years in Medicine,* and the school's two extant catalogues at the National Library of Medicine.

47. *JAMA* 59 (1912): 639.

48. W. P. Thirkield to H. S. Pritchett, February 21, 1910, Flexner Papers, Library of Congress.

49. [E. A. Balloch] to W. P. Thirkield, May 16, 1910, CFAT-Howard University Files, Carnegie Foundation Archives (hereafter cited as CFA), New York.

50. W. P. Thirkield to A. Carnegie, October 31, 1910, Carnegie Corporation (hereafter cited as CC)-Howard University Files, CFA.

51. [A. Carnegie] to O. G. Villard, December 9, 1910, CC-Howard University Files, CFA.

52. W. P. Thirkield to J. Bartram, May 9, 1911, CC-Howard University Files, CFA.

53. See letters in CC-Howard University Files, CFA, for 1911–1920.

54. J. Bartram to H. S. Pritchett, May 10, 1911; Pritchett to G. W. Hubbard, May 11, 1911; Hubbard to Pritchett, Jan. 4, 1913; all in CC-Meharry Files, CFA.

55. A. Carnegie to H. S. Pritchett, Dec. 9, 1914, CC-Meharry Files, CFA.

56. See letters for this decade in both the CC and CFAT Files at CFA and the GEB Papers at RA.

57. "Conditional Appropriation to Shaw University," Feb. 1, 1910, GEB Papers, Box 103, Folder 930, RAC.

58. Minutes of Council on Medical Education, June 21, 1914, p. 156, AMA Office of Medical Education, Chicago.

59. Ibid., Feb. 24, 1914, pp. 109, 224.

60. See annual education issues of *JAMA* for this decade; for example: 63 (1914): 671; 65 (1915): 704; 67 (1916): 605; see also G. W. Hubbard to H. S. Pritchett, Jan. 29, 1915, CFAT-Meharry Files, CFA.

61. *JAMA* 65 (1915): 704.

62. See, for example, A. Flexner to E. A. Balloch, Oct. 6 and Oct. 24, 1914, GEB Papers, Box 28, Folder 256; and E. C. Sage to W. C. McNeill, Feb. 8, 1915, GEB Papers, Box 28; Folder 257, RAC.

63. A. Flexner to H. S. Pritchett, Dec. 5, 1916; Pritchett to Flexner, Dec. 12, 1916; Flexner to Pritchett, Jan. 27, 1917; G. W. Hubbard to Flexner, Nov. 28, 1917; E. C. Sage to Hubbard, Dec. 10, 1917; Flexner to Pritchett, Dec. 9, 1918; all in GEB Papers, Box 133, Folder 1227, RAC.

64. A. Flexner to G. W. Hubbard, Dec. 16, 1914; Flexner to A. D. Bevan, Feb. 8, 1915; in GEB Papers, Box 133, Folder 1227, RAC. For a discussion of Flexner's position on "flexible standards" for black and southern medical schools, see D. M. Fox, "Abraham Flexner's Unpublished Report: Foundations and Medical Education, 1909–1928," *Bulletin of the History of Medicine* 54 (1980): 488–89.

65. G. W. Hubbard to E. C. Sage, Nov. 20, 1917, GEB Papers, Box 133, Folder 1227, RAC.

66. A copy of this appeal, "Crisis in Negro Medical Schools," dated Nov. 20, 1917, may be found in the Royster Family Papers, Folder "1915–1920," Southern Historical Collection, University of North Carolina at Chapel Hill. See also, S. M. Newman to A. Flexner, Jan. 14, 1918, GEB Papers, Box 702, Folder 7220, and petition dated Dec. 30, 1917 enclosed with that letter, RAC.

67. N. P. Colwell to G. N. Brink, Feb. 23, 1918, GEB Papers, Box 702, Folder 7220, RAC.

68. N. P. Colwell to H. S. Pritchett, March 12, 1918, CFAT-AMA Files, CFA; Colwell to E. C. Sage, March 15, 1918, GEB Papers, Box 702, Folder 7220, RAC.

69. See enclosure with G. N. Brink to E. C. Sage, March 11, 1918, GEB Papers, Box 702, Folder 7220, RAC.

70. H. S. Pritchett to N. P. Colwell, April 3, 1918, CFAT-AMA Files, CFA.

71. A. McD. Moore to A. Flexner, May 22, 1918, GEB Papers, Box 702, Folder 7220, RAC. See also Palmetto Medical Association of South Carolina to E. C. Sage, April 25, 1918, and W. T. B. Williams to W. Buttrick, May 13, 1918, GEB Papers, Box 702, Folder 7220, RAC.

72. A. Flexner to H. D. Arnold, May 29, 1918; Flexner to N. P. Colwell, May 29, 1918; Colwell to Flexner, May 31, 1918; GEB Papers, Box 702, Folder 7220, RAC.

73. A. Flexner to N. P. Colwell, May 29, 1918, Box 702, Folder 7220, RAC.

74. A. McD. Moore to G. N. Brink, Aug. 12, 1918, GEB Papers, Box 702, Folder 7220; "Memorandum Regarding Negro Medical Schools," Aug. 28, 1918, GEB Papers, Box 133, Folder 1228, both at RAC.

75. [H. S. Pritchett?] to Bishop Nicholson, Feb. 24, 1919, and W. Buttrick to Nicholson, March 3, 1919, GEB Papers, Box 133, Folder 1228, RAC.

76. P. Bartsch to H. S. Pritchett, April 11, 1919; Pritchett to Bartsch, April 14, 1919; both in CFAT Files, CFA; A. Flexner to Pritchett, April 27, 1921, Flexner Papers, Library of Congress.

77. Hine, "The Pursuit of Professional Equality," p. 173.

78. R. B. Fosdick, *Adventure in Giving: The Story of the General Education Board* (New York: Harper & Row, 1962), pp. 177–85; Summerville, *Educating Black Doctors,* pp. 60–105; Morais, *History of the Negro in Medicine,* pp. 92–94.

79. A. Flexner to A. P. Stokes, "Memorandum on Medical Education," Feb. 17, 1920, in Anson Phelps Stokes Papers, Addition, Series III, Box 76, Yale University Library.

80. Fosdick, *Adventure in Giving,* pp. 174–77; Logan, *Howard University,* pp. 256–57, 370–75; Morais, *History of the Negro in Medicine,* pp. 90–92.

81. H. E. Walker, *The Negro in the Medical Profession* (Charlottesville: Phelps-Stokes Fellowship Papers, University of Virginia, 1949), pp. 24–29; Morais, *History of the Negro in Medicine,* p. 94.

NOTES FOR CHAPTER 6

1. There is no discussion of osteopathic medical education in the two most recent major works. See K. Ludmerer, *Learning to Heal: The Development of American Medical Education* (New York: Basic Books, 1985); and W. G. Rothstein, *American Medical Schools and the Practice of Medicine* (New York: Oxford University Press, 1987).

2. N. Gevitz, *The D.O.s: Osteopathic Medicine in America* (Baltimore: Johns Hopkins University Press, 1982), pp. 1–47.

3. S. Hahnemann, *The Organon of Medicine,* 2d. American ed. (New York: Radde, 1843).

4. W. Beach, *The American Practice of Medicine* (New York: By the author, 1833).

5. Minutes of the Dec. 28, 1908 Meeting of the AMA CME, Archives of the American Medical Association, Chicago.

6. A. Flexner, *Medical Education in the United States and Canada* (New York: Carnegie Foundation for the Advancement of Teaching, 1910), pp. 156–58.

7. Ibid., p. 164.

8. Ibid., pp. 164–65.

9. Ibid., p. 166.

10. "The Report of the Carnegie Foundation," *Journal of Osteopathy* 17 (1910): 1192.

11. See Gevitz, *The D.O.s,* pp. 48–60.

12. "Carnegie Foundation Report," *Journal of the American Osteopathic Association* 9 (1910): 500–03.

13. "Report of the Committee on Education," *Journal of the American Osteopathic Association* 10 (1910): 35–38.

14. H. Weiskotten et. al., *Medical Education in the United States, 1934–1939* (Chicago: AMA, 1940), pp. 15, 67.

15. Ibid., p. 107.

16. See Gevitz, *The D.O.s*, pp. 79–81.

17. G. A. Laughlin, "Hindrances to Osteopathic Progress," *Journal of the American Osteopathic Association* 31 (1932): 519.

18. R. H. Singleton, "Report of the Committee on American Osteopathic Foundation," *Journal of the American Osteopathic Association* 31 (1932): 511.

19. Gevitz, *The D.O.s*, p. 80.

20. Ibid., pp. 80–81.

21. S. L. Baker, "Physician Licensure Laws in the United States, 1865–1915," *Journal of the History of Medicine* 39 (1984): 173–97.

22. Minutes of the Joint Councils on Medical Education, Oct. 25, 1907. Bound with minutes of the AMA CME, Archives of the American Medical Association, Chicago. See also R. L. Thomas, "Our Future," *Eclectic Medical Journal* 68 (1908): 645–47.

23. This conclusion is based upon a reading of the AMA CME minutes of meetings between 1907 and 1928, which contain summaries of on-site inspections. For Marxist interpretations see E. R. Brown, *Rockefeller Medical Men* (Berkeley: University of California Press, 1979), pp. 135–58; and H. S. Berliner, "A Larger Perspective on the Flexner Report," *International Journal of Health Services* 5 (1975): 573–92.

24. "Classification of Medical Schools," *JAMA* 61 (1913): 585–87.

25. Data derived from "Medical Education in the United States," *JAMA* 79 (1922): 629–33.

26. Ibid., and Flexner, *Medical Education*, pp. 329–35.

27. Flexner, *Medical Education*, pp. 329–35.

28. See W. G. Rothstein, *American Physicians in the Nineteenth Century: From Sects to Science* (Baltimore: Johns Hopkins University Press, 1972), pp. 298–326; M. Kaufman, *Homeopathy in America: The Rise and Fall of a Medical Heresy* (Baltimore: Johns Hopkins University Press, 1971), pp. 156–73.

29. See the AMA CME minutes for Feb. 24, 1914; Inspection of Hahnemann Medical College and Hospital, Chicago, dated Jan. 16, 1917 in the minutes; and CME minutes dated March 2, 1924.

30. Ohio State University established a homeopathic college in 1914. For a portrait of this short-lived institution see W. H. Roberts, "Orthodoxy vs. Homeopathy: Ironic Developments Following the Flexner Report at the Ohio State University," *Bulletin of the History of Medicine* 60 (1986): 73–87.

31. Kaufman, *Homeopathy in America*, p. 177.

32. Rothstein, *American Physicians*, p. 296.

33. Gevitz, *The D.O.s*, p. 50.

34. Data culled from Flexner, *Medical Education*, pp. 329–35; "Medical Education in the United States," 87 (1926): 570; and Gevitz, *The D.O.s*, p. 149.

35. Data culled from Flexner, *Medical Education*, pp. 329–35.

36. Morris Fishbein, *The Medical Follies* (New York: Boni and Liveright, 1925), p. 54.

37. F. Etherington and S. S. Ryerson, "Preliminary Report to the Joint Advisory Committee Representing the College of Physicians and Surgeons of Ontario, the Ontario Medical Association, and the Universities in Ontario Engaged in the Teaching of Medicine on Osteopathic Colleges and Teaching in Kirksville,

Philadelphia, Des Moines, and Chicago," dated March 1, 1934, microfilmed, Archives of the American Osteopathic Association, Chicago.

38. N. Gevitz, " 'A Coarse Sieve': Basic Science Boards and Medical Licensure in the United States," *Journal of the History of Medicine* 43 (1988): 36–63.

39. Gevitz, *The D.O.s*, p. 84.

40. Ibid., pp. 84–85.

41. Ibid., p. 85.

42. Ibid., pp. 85–86.

43. Ibid., pp. 86–87.

44. Ibid., pp. 130–36.

NOTES FOR CHAPTER 7

1. O. W. Anderson, *Health Services in the United States, A Growth Enterprise Since 1875* (Chicago: University of Chicago Press, 1985), pp. 13–23.

2. O. W. Anderson and N. Gevitz, "The General Hospital," in *Handbook of Health, Health Care and the Health Professions,* ed D. Mechanic (New York: The Free Press, 1982), pp. 308–13.

3. A. Flexner, *I Remember* (New York: Simon and Schuster, 1940), p. 75.

4. A. Flexner, *Medical Education in the United States and Canada* (New York: Carnegie Foundation, 1910).

5. See, for example R. Stevens, *In Sickness and in Wealth* (New York: Basic Books, 1989), pp. 17–51, 284–320.

6. P. Starr, The Social Transformation of American Medicine (New York: Basic Books, 1982), pp. 261–65.

7. I. S. Falk, M. C. Klem, and N. Sinai, *The Incidence of Illness and the Receipt and Costs of Medical Care Among Representative Families; Experiences in Twelve Consecutive Months During 1928–1931,* Committee on the Costs of Medical Care no. 26 (Chicago: University of Chicago Press, 1933).

8. R. I. Lee and L. W. Jones, *The Fundamentals of Medical Care: An Outline of the Fundamentals of Good Medical Care and an Estimate of the Service Required to Supply the Medical Needs of the United States,* Committee on the Costs of Medical Care no. 22 (Chicago: University of Chicago Press, 1933).

9. D. Neuhauser, *Coming of Age: A 52-Year History of the American College of Hospital Administrators and of Profession It Serves, 1933–1983* (Chicago: Pluribus Press, 1983), p. 12.

10. O. W. Anderson, "The History of the Graduate Program in Hospital Administration at the University of Chicago: A Case of Dynamic Marginality," *Journal of Health Administration Education* 3 (Spring 1985, Part II): 5–25.

11. G. L. Filerman, "The Development and Current Status of Programs in Health Administration," *Journal of Health Administration Education* 3 (Spring 1985, Part II): 83–92.

12. W. Rothstein, *American Medical Schools and the Practice of Medicine* (New York: Oxford University Press, 1987), pp. 283–86.

13. N. Sinai, M. F. Hall, and R. E. Holmes, *Medical Relief Administration: A Final Report of the Experience in Essex County, Ontario* (Windsor Ontario: Essex County Medical Society, 1939).

14. O. Peterson et al., *An Analytical Study of North Carolina General Practice, 1953–1954* (Evanston, Illinois: Association of American Medical Colleges, 1956).

15. K. Clute, *The General Practitioner: A Study of Medical Education and Practice in Ontario and Nova Scotia* (Toronto: University of Toronto Press, 1963).

16. R. Andersen and O. W. Anderson, *A Decade of Health Services: Social Survey Trends in Use and Expenditure* (Chicago: University of Chicago Press, 1967), p. 33.

17. O. W. Anderson et al., *HMO Development: Patterns and Prospects—A Comparative Analysis of HMOs* (Chicago: Pluribus Press, 1985), p. 2.

18. M. Garg, R. Rabidoux and J. Feinglass, "Medical Care Inflation and Government Cost Containment Policies, 1966 to 1983," in *The Medicare System of Prospective Payment*, ed. M. Garg and B. Barzansky (New York: Praeger, 1986), pp. 7–9.

19. D. Palmer, "Professional Review Organizations," in *The Medicare System*, p. 64.

20. M. R. Chasen et al., "Variations in the Use of Medical and Surgical Services by the Medicare Population," *The New England Journal of Medicine* 314 (1986): 285–90. This article is an example of many on the same topic.

21. J. Wennberg, "Which Rate is Right?" *The New England Journal of Medicine* 314 (1986): 310–11.

22. A. Donabedian, *The Definition of Quality and Approaches to Its Assessment. Volume I—Explorations in Quality Assessment and Monitoring* (Ann Arbor, Michigan: Health Administration Press, 1980).

23. R. Greene, *Assuring Quality in Medical Care: The State of the Art* (Cambridge, Massachusetts: Ballinger, 1976).

24. O. W. Anderson and M. C. Shields, "Quality Measurement and Control in Physician Decision Making: State of the Art," *Health Services Research* 17 (1982): 125–55.

25. Yankelovich, Skelly and White, Inc. *Summary Report* (Emmaus, Pennsylvania: Rodale Press, 1983).

26. See Chapter 11 in this volume by Kindig and Movassaghi for a discussion of physician manpower.

27. P. Starr, *The Social Transformation of American Medicine* (New York, Basic Books, 1982), p. 428. Starr believes the profession is encountering a private bureaucracy as well as a public one.

28. Graduate Program in Health Administration, University of Chicago, Twenty-eighth Annual George Bugbee Symposium on Hospital Affairs, "Cost Containment and Physician Autonomy: Implications for Quality of Care" (Chicago, Center for Health Administration Studies, 1987).

29. Comment by W. R. Scott in "Issues and Discussion of Chapter 15," in *Organization Research on Health Institutions*, ed. B. Georgopolis (Ann Arbor, Michigan: Institute for Social Research, 1972), p. 388.

NOTES FOR CHAPTER 8

1. J. R. Schofield, *New and Expanded Medical Schools, Mid-Century to the 1980s* (San Francisco: Jossey Bass, 1984).

2. Ibid., p. 15.

3. R. Stevens, *American Medicine and the Public Interest* (New Haven: Yale University Press, 1971), p. 352.

4. W. G. Rothstein, *American Medical Schools and the Practice of Medicine* (New York: Oxford University Press, 1987), p. 237.

5. Stevens, *American Medicine*, p. 363.

6. R. Fein and G. Weber, *Financing Medical Education* (New York: McGraw Hill Book Company, 1971), p. 58.

7. AMA, "Medical Education in the United States," *JAMA*, 178 (1961): 587.

8. Fein and Weber, *Financing Medical Education*, p. 59.

9. Rothstein, *American Medical Schools*, p. 238.

10. Ibid., p. 248 notes that in 1961–62, approximately one-third of the basic science faculty and one-quarter of clinical faculty received all or part of their salaries from federal sources. In 1970–71, approximately one-half of all faculty received such funding.

11. Sponsored research funds were not distributed evenly across schools, as evidenced by the fact that roughly one-third of accredited medical schools received some 74 percent of biomedical research funding throughout the late 1960s and 1970s (Schofield, *New and Expanded Medical Schools*, p. 133). Thus, for some institutions, the impact of biomedical research funding was felt only indirectly as a general shift in the educational climate to one which emphasized the pursuit of research to a greater extent than previously.

12. Stevens, *American Medicine*, p. 349.

13. P. J. Feldstein, *Health Associations and the Demand for Legislation: The Political Economy of Health* (Cambridge: Ballinger Publishing Company, 1977), p. 62.

14. Stevens, *American Medicine*, p. 365.

15. For an overview of federal health manpower and training programs see S. P. Korper, "Federal Health Manpower Legislation: History and Prologue," In *Medical Education Financing*, ed. J. Hadley (New York: Prodist, 1980), pp. 278–92.

16. AAMC, *Federal Support of Medical School Programs* (Washington, D.C., AAMC, 1982), p. 6.

17. J. Iglehart, "Federal Support of Health Manpower Education," *New England Journal of Medicine* 314 (1986): 324–28.

18. A. Crowley, "Highlights of the 1987 Education Issue," *JAMA* 258 (1987): 1005–06.

19. L. Lewin and R. A. Berzon, "Health Professions Education: State Responsibilities Under the New Federalism," *Health Affairs* 1 (1982): 69–85.

20. For a more complete discussion of the impact of federal health manpower programs on the supply of physicians, see Chapter 11 in this volume by Kindig and Movassaghi.

21. AAMC, Committee on the Financing of Medical Education, "Financing Undergraduate Medical Education," *Journal of Medical Education* 49 (Supplement, November, 1974): 1091–111; Rothstein, *American Medical Schools*, 287.

22. G. K. MacLeod and M. R. Schwarz, "Faculty Practice Plans: Profile and Critiques," *JAMA* 256 (1986): 59; Rothstein, *American Medical Schools*, p. 260.

23. MacLeod and Schwarz, "Faculty Practice Plans," pp. 58–62.

24. Ibid. Note that the number of full-time clinical faculty in the nation's medical schools increased from 28,602 in 1975–76 to 44,984 in 1984–85.

25. Rothstein, *American Medical Schools,* p. 263.

26. L. Cluff, "Responsibility, Accountability, and Self-Discipline: Changing Emphases in Medical Education," *The Pharos* 44 (Winter): 2–5.

27. R. Petersdorf, "The Scylla and Charybdis of Medical Education," *Journal of Medical Education* 63 (1988): 88–93; Rothstein, *American Medical Schools,* p. 261.

28. R. Jones, M. Mirsky, and J. Keyes, "Clinical Practice of Medical School Faculties: An AAMC Survey of Problems and Issues," *Journal of Medical Education* 60 (1985): 909.

29. Ibid., p. 905.

30. C. Schmidt, P. Zieve, and B. D'Lugoff, "A Practice Plan in a Municipal Teaching Hospital," *The New England Journal of Medicine* 304 (1981): 268; D. Rogers and R. Blendon, "The Academic Medical Center Today," *Annals of Internal Medicine* 100 (1984): 754.

31. Petersdorf, "The Scylla and Charybdis," p. 92.

32. Rothstein, *American Medical Schools,* p. 268.

33. Jones, Mirsky, and Keyes, "Clinical Practice of Medical School Faculties," p. 900; Petersdorf, "The Scylla and Charybdis," p. 91; Rogers and Blendon, "The Academic Medical Center Today," p. 754.

34. F. Guggenheim and C. Nadelson, "Earn-As-You-Go Pressures in Academic Psychiatry," *American Journal of Psychiatry* 141 (1984): 1571–73.

35. Rogers and Blendon, "The Academic Medical Center Today," p. 752.

36. Jones, Mirsky, and Keyes, "Clinical Practice of Medical School Faculties," pp. 897–910; P. Plumeri, "Must We Pay for Medical Education?" *Journal of Clinical Gastroenterology* 17 (1985): 93–96; Schmidt, Zieve, and D'Lugoff, "A Practice Plan," p. 268.

37. Jones, Mirsky, and Keyes, "Clinical Practice of Medical School Faculties," pp. 897–910.

38. E. Stemmler, "Faculty Practice in Academic Centers," *Journal of Medical Education* 60 (1985): 949–50.

39. Jones, Mirsky, and Keyes, "Clinical Practice of Medical School Faculties," p. 907.

40. Stemmler, "Faculty Practice," p. 949.

41. Fein and Weber, *Financing Medical Education,* p. 211.

42. MacLeod and Schwarz, "Faculty Practice Plans," pp. 58–62.

43. Cluff, "Responsibilities, Accountability, and Self-Discipline," p. 4.

NOTES FOR CHAPTER 9

1. K. Ludmerer, *Learning to Heal* (New York: Basic Books, Inc., 1985), pp. 152–54.

2. W. Osler, "The Natural Method of Teaching the Subject of Medicine," *JAMA* 36 (1901): 1673–75.

3. V. Vaughan, "Reorganization of Clinical Teaching," *JAMA* 64 (1915): 786–87.

4. G. Dock, "The Student's Clinical Course in Medicine," *American Medical Association Bulletin* 13 (1917): 132–33.

5. W. Rothstein, *American Medical Schools and the Practice of Medicine* (New York: Oxford University Press, 1987), p. 126.

6. Ibid., pp. 171–72.

7. Commission on Medical Education, *Final Report* (New York: Office of the Director of the Study, 1932), pp. 203, 210.

8. Ibid., pp. 209–10.

9. H. Weiskotten et al., *Medical Education in the United States, 1934–1939* (Chicago: American Medical Association, 1940), pp. 177, 185, 189–90.

10. J. Deitrick and R. Berson, *Medical Schools in the United States at Mid-Century* (New York: McGraw Hill, 1953), pp. 235–36.

11. Ibid., pp. 248–50; W. Wiggins, "A Consideration of Preceptorial Medical Education in the United States," *Journal of Medical Education* 32 (1957): 118.

12. D. Anderson, F. Manlove, and A. Tipner, "Medical Education in the United States and Canada," *JAMA* 147 (1951): 150; E. Turner et al., "Medical Education in the United States and Canada," *JAMA* 156 (1954): 580.

13. Wiggins, "Preceptorial Medical Education," p. 120.

14. C. Lewis, R. Fein, and D. Mechanic, *A Right to Health* (New York: John Wiley and Sons, 1976), p. 63.

15. J. Rising, "The Rural Preceptorship," *The Journal of the Kansas Medical Society* (March 1962): 81–82.

16. J. Verby, "The Minnesota Rural Physician Associate Program for Medical Students," *Journal of Medical Education* 63 (1988): 427–31.

17. J. D. Voorhees, M. Bennett, and A. Counsellor, in *Implementing Problem-Based Medical Education,* ed. A. Kaufman (New York: Springer Publishing Company, 1985), p. 124–25.

18. Wiggins, "Preceptorial Medical Education," p. 120.

19. Deitrick and Berson, *Medical Schools in the United States,* p. 256; Rothstein, *American Medical Schools and the Practice of Medicine,* p. 308.

20. See, for example, Voorhees, Bennett, and Counsellor in *Implementing Problem-Based Medical Education,* pp. 127–29.

21. P. Snoke and E. Weinerman, "Comprehensive Care Programs in University Medical Centers," *Journal of Medical Education* 40 (1965): 627.

22. Rothstein, *American Medical Schools and the Practice of Medicine,* pp. 308–9.

23. Snoke and Weinerman, "Comprehensive Care Programs," p. 627; P. Kendall and G. Reader, "Innovations in Medical Education of the 1950s Contrasted with Those of the 1970s and 1980s," *Journal of Health and Social Behavior* 29 (1988): 283.

24. P. Lee, *Medical Schools and the Changing Times* (Evanston, Illinois: Association of American Medical Colleges, 1962), pp. 32–34.

25. Snoke and Weinerman, "Comprehensive Care Programs," p. 633.

26. Lee, *Medical Schools and the Changing Times,* pp. 39–44; Snoke and Weinerman, "Comprehensive Care Programs," pp. 630–33.

27. Rothstein, *American Medical Schools and the Practice of Medicine,* p. 309.

28. E. Saward in *Health Maintenance Organizations and Academic Medical Centers,* ed. J. Hudson and H. Nevins (Menlo Park, California: Henry J. Kaiser Family Foundation, 1981), p. 25.

29. S. Schroeder, S. Werner, and T. Piemme, "Primary Care in the Academic Medical Centers: A Report of a Survey by the AAMC," *Journal of Medical Education* 49 (1974): 826–27.

30. J. Isaacs and M. Madoff, "Undergraduate Medical Education in Prepaid Health Care Plan Settings," *Journal of Medical Education* 59 (1984): 618–19.

31. R. Hoft and R. Glaser, "The Problems and Benefits of Associating Academic Medical Centers with Health Maintenance Organizations," *New England Journal of Medicine* 307 (1982): 1686–87; II. Kirz, "Costs and Benefits of Medical Student Training to a Health Maintenance Organization," *JAMA* 256 (1986): 734–39.

32. Schroeder, Werner, and Piemme, "Primary Care in the Academic Medical Centers," p. 824.

33. J. Giacolone and J. Hudson, "Primary Care Trends in U.S. Medical Schools and Teaching Hospitals," *Journal of Medical Education* 52 (1977): 972–73.

34. *1989–90 Curriculum Directory* (Washington, D.C.: Association of American Medical Colleges, 1989), pp. T2-T3.

35. Unpublished data from the 1988–89 Liaison Committee on Medical Education Annual Medical School Questionnaire, American Medical Association, Chicago, Illinois.

36. G. Rosevear and N. Gary, "Changes in Admissions, Lengths of Stay, and Discharge Diagnoses at a Major University-Affiliated Teaching Hospital: Implications for Medical Education," *Academic Medicine* 64 (1989): 253–58; S. Schroeder, "Expanding the Site of Clinical Education: Moving Beyond the Hospital Walls," *Journal of General Internal Medicine* 3 (Supplement 1988): S8-S10.

37. G. Moore, "Health Maintenance Organizations and Medical Education: Breaking the Barriers," *Academic Medicine* 65 (1990): 428–29; J. Wooliscroft and T. Schwenk, "Teaching and Learning in the Ambulatory Setting," *Academic Medicine* 64 (1989): 645–46.

38. J. Garrard and J. Verby, "Comparisons of Medical Student Experiences in Rural and University Settings," *Journal of Medical Education* 52 (1977): 807–10.

39. Moore, "Health Maintenance Organizations," pp. 429–30; G. Perkoff, "Teaching Clinical Medicine in the Ambulatory Setting: An Idea Whose Time May Have Finally Come," *New England Journal of Medicine* 314 (1986): 29.

NOTES FOR CHAPTER 10

1. See, for example, P. Starr, *The Social Transformation of American Medicine* (New York: Basic Books, 1982), pp. 17–21.

2. H. S. Berliner, *A System of Scientific Medicine* (New York: Tavistock Publications, 1985), see, especially pp. 1–6, 111–117. E. Riska and P. Vinten-Johansen, "The Involvement of the Behavioral Sciences in American Medicine," *International Journal of Health Services* 11 (1981): 583–96.

3. J. R. Scofield *New and Expanded Medical Schools: Mid-Century to the 1980s* (San Francisco: Jossey-Bass, Inc., 1984), pp. 5–8, 320–61.

4. A. Flexner, *Medical Education in the United States and Canada* (New York: Carnegie Foundation, 1910).

5. E. R. Brown, *Rockefeller Medicine Men: Medicine and Capitalism in America* (Berkeley: University of California Press, 1979) pp. 135–91; K. Ludmerer, *Learning to Heal: The Development of American Medical Education* (New York: Basic Books, 1985) pp. 191–206.

6. Commission on Medical Education, *Final Report* (New York: Office of the Director of the Study, 1932); H. G. Weiskotten et al., *Medical Education in the United States, 1934–1939* (Chicago: American Medical Association, 1940); J. E. Deitrick and R. C. Berson, Medical Schools in the United States at Mid-Century (Evanston: Association of American Medical Colleges, 1960). L. T. Coggeshall, *Planning for Medical Progress Through Education* (Evanston, Illinois: Association of American Medical Colleges, 1965).

7. AMA CME, *Future Directions for Medical Education* (Chicago: American Medical Association, 1982); *Physicians for the Twenty-First Century* (Washington, D.C.: AAMC, 1984); *The New Biology and Medical Education,* ed. C. P. Friedman and E. F. Purcell (New York: Josiah Macy, Jr. Foundation, 1985); *Clinical Education and the Doctor of Tomorrow,* ed. B. Gastel and D. Rogers (New York: The New York Academy of Medicine, 1989).

8. Scofield, *New and Expanded Medical Schools,* pp. 19–28.

9. G. Williams, *Western Reserve's Experiment in Medical Education and Its Outcome* (New York: Oxford University Press, 1980); *Medical Education Since 1960: Marching to a Different Drummer,* ed. A. Hunt and L. Weeks, (East Lansing: Michigan State Foundation, 1979), pp. 235–58, 321–38.

10. S. Schroeder, J. Showstack, and T. Gerber, "Residency Training in Internal Medicine: Time for a Change?' " *Annals of Internal Medicine* 104 (1986): 554–61.

11. Ibid.

12. D. Kindig and S. Lastiri, "Administrative Medicine: A New Medical Specialty?" *Health Affairs* 5 (Winter 1986): 146–56.

13. D. Baldwin and M. Baldwin, "Interdisciplinary Education and Health Team Training: A Model for Learning and Service," in *Medical Education Since 1960,* pp. 190–221.

14. American Board of Medical Specialties, *Annual Report and Reference Handbook–1991* (Evanston: ABMS, 1991), p. 23.

15. W. Graves, "Some Factors Tending Toward Adequate Instruction in Nervous and Mental Diseases," *JAMA* 63 (1914): 1701–13.

16. T. Webster, "Psychiatry and Behavioral Science Curriculum Time in United States Schools of Medicine and Osteopathy," *Journal of Medical Education* 42: 690.

17. Group for the Advancement of Psychiatry, *The Preclinical Teaching of Psychiatry,* Report 54 (New York: Group for the Advancement of Psychiatry, 1962); Webster, "Psychiatry and Behavioral Sciences Curriculum Time," p. 687–96.

18. ABMS, *Annual Report–1991,* p. 27.

19. See, for example, S. Jonas and S. Rosenberg, "Ambulatory Care," in *Health Care Delivery in the United States, 3rd edn.,* S. Jonas ed. (New York: Springer Publishing Company, 1986), pp. 153–54.

20. J. R. Scofield, *New and Expanded Medical Schools,* pp. 262–65.

21. 1992–93 Medical School Admission Requirements (Washington, D.C.: AAMC, 1991 pp. 380–408; see, for example, E. G. Dimond, "The UMKC Medical Education Experiment," *JAMA* 260 (1988): 956–58.

22. R. Ebert and E. Ginzberg, "The Reform of Medical Education," *Health Affairs* 7 (Supplement 1988): 5–38.

23. *Assessing Clinical Competence,* ed. V. Neufeld and G. Norman (New York:

Springer Publishing Company, 1985); J. D. Hamilton, "The McMaster Curriculum: A Critique," *British Medical Journal* 1 (1976): 1191–96; P. Stillman, M. Regan, and D. Swanson, "A Diagnostic Fourth-Year Performance Assessment," *Archives of Internal Medicine* 147 (1987): 1981–85; Stillman, Regan, and Swanson, "Ensuring the Clinical Competence of Medical School Graduates Through Standardized Patients," *Archives of Internal Medicine* 147 (1987): 1049–52; H. Barrows, R. Williams, and R. Moy, "A Comprehensive Performance-Based Assessment of Fourth-Year Students' Clinical Skills," *Journal of Medical Education* 62 (1987): 805–09; N. Black and R. Harden, "Providing Feedback to Students on Clinical Skills Using the Objective Structured Clinical Examination," *Medical Education* 20 (1986): 48–52; D. Elliot and D. Hickam, "Evaluation of Physical Examination Skills," *JAMA* 258 (1987): 3405–08.

24. P. Stillman et al., "A Diagnostic Fourth-Year Performance Assessment," *Archives of Internal Medicine* 147 (1987): 1981–85.

25. *Implementing Problem-Based Medical Education: Lessons from Successful Innovations,* ed. A. Kaufman, (New York: Springer, 1985); P. Ways, F. Loftus, and J. Jones, "Focal Problem Teaching in Medical Education," *Journal of Medical Education* 48 (1973): 565.

26. D. C. Tosteson et al., "A New Pathway for General Medical Education," *Harvard Medical Alumni Bulletin* (Winter 1984): 14–24.

27. M. Kantrowitz et al., *Innovative Tracks in Established Health Science Institutions: Strategies for Relevant Change* (Geneva: World Health Organization, 1987), pp. 73–232.

28. D. Baldwin and M. Baldwin, "Interdisciplinary Education and Health Team Training," in *Medical Education Since 1960,* pp. 190–221.

29. D. Bok, "Needed: A New Way to Train Doctors," *Harvard Magazine* (May-June, 1984): 32–71; J. Alpert and R. Coles, "Premedical Education," *Archives of Internal Medicine* 147 (1987): 633–34.

30. D. Kennedy, E. Pattishall, and C. Fletcher, *Teaching Behavioral Sciences in Schools of Medicine, Summary Report.* National Center for Health Services Research, vol. 1, 1972-reprint. (Baltimore, Maryland: Association for Behavioral Sciences and Medical Education, 1983); *Behavioral Sciences and Medical Education: A Report of Four Conferences,* #NIH–72–41 (Washington, D.C.: National Institutes of Health, 1972).

31. A. Somers, "Four 'Orphan' Areas in Current Medical Education: What Hope for Adoption?" *Family Medicine* 19 (1987): 137–40.

32. J. P. Hubbard, *Measuring Medical Education,* 2nd ed. (Philadelphia: Lea and Febiger, 1978), p. 9.

33. D. Kennedy, E. Pattishall, and D. Baldwin, *Medical Education and the Behavioral Sciences,* ABSAME no. 83–02 (Baltimore: Association for the Behavioral Sciences and Medical Education, 1983)

34. D. Rogers, "Medical Academe and the Problems of Health Care Provisions," *Archives of Internal Medicine* 135 (1975): 364–69.

35. J. Rest, "Can Ethics be Taught in Professional Schools," *The Psychological Researcher* (Winter 1988): 22–26.

36. J. Sheehan et al., "Moral Judgment as a Predictor of Clinical Performance," *Evaluation and the Health Professions* 3 (1980): 393–404.

37. D. Self, F. Wolinsky, and D. Baldwin, "The Effect of Teaching Medical

Ethics on Medical Students' Moral Reasoning," *Academic Medicine* 64 (1989): 755–59.

38. L. Osborne and C. Martin, "The Importance of Listening to Medical Students' Experiences When Teaching Them Medical Ethics," *Journal of Medical Ethics* 15 (1989): 35–38.

39. Stillman, Regan, and Swanson, "Ensuring the Clinical Competence of Medical School Graduates," pp. 1949–52; Barrows, Williams, and Moy, "A Comprehensive Performance-Based Assessment," pp. 805–09.

40. P. Small, "Basic Science Education: Problems and Possible Improvements," in *The New Biology and Medical Education*, pp. 211–20.

41. J. Todd, "Perspectives: The American Medical Association," *Health Affairs* 7 (Supplement 1988): 83–86.

42. Ebert and Ginzberg, "The Reform of Medical Education," pp. 5–39.

43. M. Bussigel, B. Barzansky, and G. Grenholm, *Innovation Processes in Medical Education* (New York: Praeger Publishing Company, 1988), pp. 121–37.

44. Ibid., pp. 138–43.

45. D. Rogers, "Some Musings on Medical Education: Is it Going Astray?" *Pharos* (Spring 1982): 11–14; K. Sheehan et al., "A Pilot Study of Medical Student 'Abuse': Student Perceptions of Mistreatment and Misconduct in Medical School," *JAMA* 263 (1990): 533–37.

46. Commission on Medical Education, *Final Report*, p. 35.

NOTES FOR CHAPTER 11

1. The Report of the Graduate Medical Education National Advisory Committee (GMENAC) vols. 1–7 USDHHS Publication Nos. (HRA) 81–651 to 81–657 (Washington, D.C.: USDHSS, 1980).

2. R. Fein, *The Doctor Shortage: An Economic Diagnosis* (Washington, D.C.: The Brookings Institution, 1967).

3. E. Ginzberg et al., "The Expanding Physician Supply and Health Policy," *Milbank Memorial Fund Quarterly/Health and Society* 59 (1981): 508–41.

4. D. McNutt, "GMENAC: Its Manpower Forecasting Framework," *American Journal of Public Health* 71 (1981): 1125.

5. I. Jacoby, "Graduate Medical Education," *JAMA* 245 (1981): 1046–51.

6. M. A. Bowman et al, "Estimates of Physician Requirements for 1990 for the Specialties of Neurology, Anesthesiology, Nuclear Medicine, Pathology, Physical Medicine and Rehabilitation, and Radiology—A Further Application of the GMENAC Methodology," *JAMA* 250 (1983): 2623–27.

7. M. A. Bowman and W. B. Walsh, Jr, "Perspectives on the GMENAC Report," *Health Affairs* 1 (1982): 55–60.

8. U. Reinhardt, "The GMENAC Forecast: An Alternative View," *American Journal of Public Health* 71 (1981): 1149.

9. R. Mounsey, "The Dark Side of GMENAC," *American College of Surgeons Bulletin* (April 1981): 10–15.

10. USDHHS, *Third Report to the President and Congress on the Status of Health Professions Personnel in the United States* (Washington, D.C.: USDHHS, 1982).

11. J. Igelhart, "Trends in Health Personnel," *Health Affairs* 5 (1986): 128–37.

12. A. Crowley et al., "Undergraduate Medical Education," *JAMA* 256 (1986): 1557.

13. M. Reich, "Undergraduate Osteopathic Medical Education," *Journal of the American Osteopathic Association* 89 (1989): 1437.

14. Crowley et al., "Undergraduate Medical Education," p. 1557.

15. D. G. Johnson et al., "United States Citizens Studying Medicine Abroad," *New England Journal of Medicine* 315 (1986): 1525–32.

16. S. S. Mick et al., "United States Foreign Medical Graduates in Connecticut," *Medical Care* 14 (1976): 489; Mick and J. Worobey, "Future Role of Foreign Medical Graduates," *U.S. Medical Practice Health Services Research* 21 (1986): 85.

17. Crowley et al., "Undergraduate Medical Education," p. 1557.

18. M. W. Smith and V. Kliner Fowkes, "Unlicensed Foreign Medical Graduates in California," *Medical Care* 21 (1983): 1168–86.

19. USDHHS, *Minorities and Women in the Health Fields* (Washington, D.C.: DHPA (Report 7–82), 1981).

20. Crowley et al., "Undergraduate Medical Education," p. 1557.

21. USDHHS, *Estimates and Projections of Black and Hispanic Physicians, Dentists, and Pharmacists to 2010.* (Washington, D.C.: USDHHS (Publication No. HRS-P-DV–1), May 1986).

22. S. N. Keith et al., "Effects of Affirmative Action in Medical Schools—A Study of the Class of 1975," *The New England Journal of Medicine* 313 (1985): 1519–25.

23. Koba Associates, *The Treatment Practices of Black Physicians*, DHEW Pub. 80–628 (Washington, D.C.: U.S. Government Printing Office, 1979).

24. J. P. Weiner et al., "Assessing a Methodology for Physician Requirement Forecasting—Replication of GMENAC's Need-based Model for the Pediatric Specialty," *Medical Care* 25 (1987): 426–36; D. M. Steinwachs et al., "A Comparison of the Requirement for Primary Care Physicians in HMOs with Projections Made by GMENAC," *The New England Journal of Medicine* 314 (1986): 217–22; J. E. Harris, "How Many Doctors are Enough," *Health Affairs* 5 (1986): 73–83.

25. American Academy of Pediatrics, Committee on Pediatric Manpower, "Critique of the Final Report of the GMENAC," *Pediatrics* 67 (1981): 585–96.

26. American Academy of Physician Assistants, *Total Physician Assistant Population* (Arlington, Virginia: AAPA, 1985).

27. R. D. Carter, D. A. Oliver, and H. B. Perry, *Secondary Analysis: 1981 National Survey of Physician Assistants*, Final Report to National Center for Health Services Research (Grant no. HS–04862) (Rockville, Maryland: USDHHS, 1984); American Academy of Physician Assistants, 1985 Master File Survey, Preliminary Report, (Arlington, Virginia: AAPA, 1985).

28. USDHHS, *Fifth Report to the President and Congress on the Status of Health Personnel in the United States*, Pub. no. HRS P-OD–86–1 Washington D.C., DHHS 1986; J. L. Weston, "Distribution of Nurse Practitioners and Physician Assistants, Implications of Legal Constraints and Reimbursement," *Public Health Reports* 95 (1980): 253–58.

29. American Academy of Physician Assistants, *Master File Survey*.

30. USDHHS, *Fifth Report*; Weston, "Distribution of Nurse Practitioners and Physician Assistants," pp. 253–58.

31. Weiner, "Physician Requirement Forecasting," pp. 426–36; Steinwachs et al., "The Requirement for Primary Care Physicians," pp. 217–22.

32. American Academy of Pediatrics, "Critique of the Final Report of the GMENAC," pp. 585–96.

33. P. P. Budetti, "The Impending Pediatric Surplus: Causes, Implications, and Alternatives," *Pediatrics* 67 (1981): 597–606.

34. H. Perry, D. E. Detmer, and D. J. Buchanan-Davidson, "Policy Proposal for Correcting the Imbalance in General Surgical Manpower," *Surgery* (1984): 243–48.

35. E. Ginzberg, "A New Physicians' Supply Policy is Needed," *JAMA* 250 (1983): 2621–22.

36. W. D. Spitzer, "The Nurse Practitioner Revisited—Slow Death of a Good Idea," *The New England Journal of Medicine* 310 (1984): 1049–51.

37. F. N. Miller, "Nurse Providers: A Resource for Growing Population Needs," *Business and Health* (1985): 38–42.

38. U. Reinhardt, *Physician Productivity and the Demand for Health Manpower: An Economic Analysis* (Cambridge, Mass.: Ballinger Publishing Company, 1975).

39. K. Davis, "Implications of an Expanding Supply of Physicians: Evidence from a Cross-Sectional Analysis," *The Johns Hopkins Medical Journal* 150 (1982): 55–64; Ginzberg, "A New Physicians Supply Policy," pp. 2621–22.

40. H. S. Luft and P. Arno, "Impact of Increasing Physician Supply: A Scenario for the Future," *Health Affairs* 5 (1986): 31–46.

41. USDHHS, *Fifth Report*.

42. M. A. Bowman and D. I. Allen, *Stress and Women Physicians* (New York: Springer-Verlag, 1985).

43. J. B. Mitchell, "Why do Women Physicians Work Fewer Hours than Men Physicians?" *Inquiry* 21 (1984): 361–68.

44. M. J. Lanska, D. Lanska, and A. A. Rimm, "Effects of Rising Percentage of Female Physicians on Projections of Physician Supply," *Journal of Medical Education* 59 (1984): 849–55.

45. A. S. Relman, "Here Come the Women," *The New England Journal of Medicine* 302 (1980): 1252.

46. Weiner et al., "Physician Requirement Forecasting," pp. 426–36.

47. A. R. Tarlov, "HMO Enrollment Growth and Physicians: The Third Compartment," *Health Affairs* 5 (1986): 23–35.

48. W. B. Schwartz, F. A. Sloan, and B. A. Mendelsonn, "Why There Will Be Little or No Physician Surplus Between Now and the Year 2000," *The New England Journal of Medicine* 318 (1988): 892.

49. D. M. Steinwachs et al., "Changing Patterns of Graduate Medical Education," *The New England Journal of Medicine* 306 (1982): 10–14; M. K. Schleiter and A. Tarlov, "National Study of Internal Medicine Manpower: VII. Internal Medicine and Fellowship Training: 1983 Update," *Annals of Internal Medicine* 99 (1983): 380–87.

50. USDHHS, *Fifth Report*; Weston, "Nurse Practitioners and Physician Assistants," pp. 253–58.

51. Bowman and Walsh, "Perspectives on the GMENAC Report," pp. 55–66.

52. D. Kindig and N. Cross-Dunham, "Physician Specialist Growth into the Twenty-First Century," *Journal of Medical Education* 60 (1985): 558–59.

53. Tarlov, "HMO Enrollment Growth and Physicians," pp. 23–35.

54. W. B. Schwartz et al., "Are We Training Too Many Subspecialists," *JAMA* 259 (1988): 233–39.

55. R. S. Stern, "Dermatologists in the Year 2000," *Archives of Dermatology* 122 (1986): 675–78.

56. J. F. Kurtzke et al., "Neurologists in the United States—Past, Present, and Future," *Neurology* 36 (1986): 1576–82.

57. M. Menken and C. G. Sheps, "Consequences of an Oversupply of Specialists—The Case of Neurology," *JAMA* 253 (1985): 1926–28.

58. S. A. Schroeder, "The Health Manpower Challenge to Internal Medicine," *Annals of Internal Medicine* 106 (1987): 768–70.

59. S. A. Schroeder, "Western European Responses to Physician Oversupply—Lesson for the United States," *JAMA* 252 (1984): 373.

60. B. S. Bloom and O. L. Peterson, "Changing the Number of Surgeons," *The New England Journal of Medicine* 303 (1980): 1227–30.

61. Perry, Detmer, and Buchanan-Davidson, "Correcting the Imbalance in General Surgical Manpower," pp. 243–48.

62. F. D. Moore, "Surgical Manpower, Past and Present Reality, Estimates for 2000," *Surgical Clinics of North America* 62 (1982): 579–602.

63. Mounsey, "The Dark Side of GMENAC," pp. 10–15.

64. AMA, *Physician Characteristics and Distribution in the United States* (Chicago: AMA, 1987).

65. W. Schwartz et al., "The Changing Geographic Distribution of Board-Certified Physicians," *The New England Journal of Medicine* 303 (1982): 1032–38.

66. J. Newhouse et al., "Where Have all the Doctors Gone," *JAMA* 247 (1982): 2392–406.

67. USDHHS, "Diffusion and the Changing Geographic Distribution of Primary Care Physicians," ODAM Report No 4–83 (Washington, D.C.: DHHS, June 1983).

68. M. A. Fruen and J. R. Cantwell, "Geographic Distribution of Physicians: Past Trends and Future Influences," *Inquiry* 19 (1982): 44–50.

69. K. Hines and N. Givner, "Physician Distribution in a Predominantly Rural State: Predictors and Trends," *Inquiry* 20 (1983): 185–90.

70. G. E. Right, *Community Characteristics and the Competition for Physicians in Rural America, 1971–1981* (Washington, D.C.: Macro Systems Inc., 1985).

71. D. L. Spencer and G. D'Elia, "The Effects of Regional Medical Education on Physician Distribution in Illinois," *Journal of Medical Education* 58 (1983): 309–15.

72. D. A. Kindig and H. Movassaghi, "The Adequacy of Physician Supply in Small Rural Counties," *Health Affairs* 8 (Summer 1989): 61–76.

73. Kindig et al., "Trends in Physician Availability in Ten Urban Areas From 1963 to 1980," *Inquiry* 24 (1987): 136–46.

74. D. A. Kindig and C. M. Taylor, "Growth in the International Physician Supply—1950 Through 1979," *JAMA* 253 (1985): 3129–32.

75. Reinhardt, *Physician Productivity and the Demand for Health Manpower*, pp. 5, 259–69.

76. Kindig and Cross-Dunham, "Physician Specialist Growth into the Twenty-First Century," pp. 558–59.

77. A. Tarlov, "The Increasing Supply of Physicians, the Changing Structure of the Health-Services System, and the Future Practice of Medicine," *The New England Journal of Medicine* 308 (1983): 1235–44.

78. Harris, "How Many Doctors are Enough," pp. 73–83.

79. Ginzberg, "A New Physicians' Supply Policy," pp. 2621–22.

80. E. Ginzberg, "The Future Supply of Physicians: From Pluralism to Policy," *Health Affairs* 1 (1982): 6–9.

81. J. Igelhart, "The Future Supply of Physicians," *The New England Journal of Medicine* 314 (1986): 860–64.

82. Schroeder, "The Health Manpower Challenge," pp. 768–70.

83. Luft and Arno, "Impact of Increasing Physician Supply," pp. 31–46.

84. M. O. Jacobs and P. D. Mott, "Physician Characteristics and Training Emphasis Considered Desirable by Leaders of HMOs," *Journal of Medical Education* 62 (1987): 725–31.

85. Tarlov, "HMO Enrollment Growth and Physicians," pp. 23–35.

86. E. P. Schloss, "Beyond GMENAC—Another Physician Shortage from 2010 to 2030?" *The New England Journal of Medicine* 318 (1988): 920; J. J. Jacobsen and A. A. Rimm, "The Projected Physician Surplus Re-evaluated," *Health Affairs* 6 (1987): 90–102.

87. D. B. Louria, "Preventing the Impending Doctor Glut," *JAMA* 250 (1983): 2603–04.

88. J. Martinsons, "U.S. M.D. Glut Limits Demand for FMG Physicians," *Hospitals* (February 1988): 67.

89. Schwartz et al., "Are we Training Too Many Medical Subspecialists?" pp. 233–39.

90. Tarlov, "HMO Enrollment Growth and Physicians," pp. 23–35.

91. W. C. Hsiao et al., "The Resource Based Relative Values," *JAMA* 260 (1988): 2347–48.

NOTES FOR CHAPTER 12

1. Commission on Medical Education, *Final Report* (New York: Office of the Director of the Study, 1932), Table 104; N. P. Colwell, "Improvements in Medical Education in Sixteen Years." *American Medical Association Bulletin* 14 (1920): 11–12.

2. A. Flexner, *Medical Education in the United States and Canada* (New York: Carnegie Foundation, 1910), p. 20.

3. See Chapter 1 in this volume by R. P. Hudson.

4. Council on Medical Education, "Proceedings of the Third Annual Conference," *JAMA* 48 (1907): 1701–07; L. King, "The Flexner Report of 1910," *JAMA* 251 (1984): 1084.

5. Flexner, *Medical Education,* p. 167.

6. W. Bierring, "Medical Licensure after Forty Years," *Federation Bulletin* 43 (1956): 107–08.

7. *Choice of a Medical School* (Chicago: Council on Medical Education, 1920), Table 2.

8. W. Rothstein, *American Medical Schools and the Practice of Medicine* (New York: Oxford University Press, 1987), p. 144.

9. D. M. Fox, "Abraham Flexner's Unpublished Report: Foundations and Medical Education 1909–1928," *Bulletin of the History of Medicine* 54 (1980): 484–85; Rothstein, *American Medical Schools,* pp. 150–51.

10. R. Stevens, *In Sickness and in Wealth* (New York: Basic Books, 1989), pp. 23–24, 28–29.

11. Rothstein, *American Medical Schools,* pp. 128–29.

12. AMA CME, *Future Directions for Medical Education* (Chicago: AMA, 1982), p. 1.

13. Ibid., pp. 2–18.

14. *Physicians for the Twenty-First Century* (Washington, D.C.: AAMC, 1984), pp. 1–2.

15. Ibid., pp. 5–22.

16. R. H. Ebert and E. Ginzberg, "The Reform of Medical Education," *Health Affairs* 7 (Supplement 1988): 6–8.

17. Ibid., pp. 34–36.

18. *Clinical Education and the Doctor of Tomorrow,* ed. B. Gastel and D. Rogers (New York: New York Academy of Medicine, 1989).

19. D. Rogers, "Clinical Education and the Doctor of Tomorrow: An Agenda for Action," in *Clinical Education and the Doctor of Tomorrow,* pp. 109–13.

20. *U.S. Medical Licensure Statistics and Current Licensure Requirements* (Chicago: AMA, 1989), pp. 1, 37.

21. H. Jonas, S. Etzel, and B. Barzansky, "Undergraduate Medical Education," *JAMA* 22 (1989): 1018.

22. See, for example, A. Kaufman et al., "The New Mexico Experiment: Educational Innovation and Institutional Change," *Academic Medicine* 64 (1989): 289.

23. See, for example, *Clinical Education and the Doctor of Tomorrow,* p. 111.

24. L. Taksel, P. Jolly, and R. Beran, "U.S. Medical School Finances," *JAMA* 262 (1989): 1023–24. Also see Chapter 8 in this volume by J. Perloff on financing undergraduate medical education.

25. See, for example, R. Ebert and E. Ginzberg, "Medical Education Reform," p. 32 and R. G. Petersdorf, "Medical Schools and Research: Is the Tail Wagging the Dog?" *Daedalus* 115 (1986): 115–17.

26. Moore, "Opening the Ambulatory Setting: Teaching Medical Students What they Need to Know." in *Clinical Education and the Doctor of Tomorrow,* pp. 81–84.

27. H. Jonas, S. Etzel, and B. Barzansky, "Undergraduate Medical Education," p. 1018.

Selected Bibliography

This Bibliography contains selected general references related to the topics in this volume. The reader is directed to the Notes for each chapter for a more comprehensive set of references for the subject.

Abraham, R., ed. *Send us a Lady Physician: Women Doctors in America, 1835–1920.* New York: W. W. Norton and Company, 1985.

Anderson, O. *Health Services in the United States, A Growth Enterprise Since 1875.* Chicago: University of Chicago Press, 1985.

Atwater, E. "Making Fewer Mistakes." *Bulletin of the History of Medicine* 57 (1983): 163–87.

Baker, S. "Physician Licensure Laws in the United States, 1865–1915. *Journal of the History of Medicine* 39 (1984): 173–97.

Berliner, H. "A Larger Perspective on the Flexner Report." *International Journal of the Health Sciences* 5 (1975): 573–92.

Berliner, H. *A System of Scientific Medicine.* New York: Tavistock Publications, 1985.

Bonner, T. *American Doctors in German Universities: A Chapter in International Intellectual Relations 1870–1914.* Lincoln: University of Nebraska Press, 1963.

Brown, E. *Rockefeller Medicine Men: Medicine and Capitalism in America.* Berkeley: University of California Press, 1979.

Burrow, J. *Organized Medicine in the Progressive Era: The Move Toward Monopoly.* Baltimore: The Johns Hopkins University Press, 1977.

Bussigel, M., B. Barzansky, and G. Grenholm, *Innovation Processes in Medical Schools.* New York: Praeger Publishing Company, 1988.

Commission on Medical Education. *Final Report.* New York: Office of the Director of the Study, 1932.

Council on Medical Education. *Future Directions for Medical Education.* Chicago: American Medical Association, 1982.

Davis, N. S. *Contributions to the History of Medical Education and Medical Institutions in the United States of America, 1776–1876.* Washington, D.C.: Government Printing Office, 1877.

Detrick, J., and R. Berson. *Medical Schools in the United States at Mid-Century*. Evanston, Illinois: Association of American Medical Colleges, 1960.

Ebert, R., and E. Ginzberg. "The Reform of Medical Education." *Health Affairs* 7 (Supplement 1988): 5–38.

Flexner, A. *An Autobiography*. New York: Simon and Schuster, 1960.

Flexner, A. *Medical Education: A Comparative Study*. New York: The Macmillan Company, 1925.

Flexner, A. *Medical Education in the United States and Canada*. New York: Carnegie Foundation, 1910.

Fox, D. "Abraham Flexner's Unpublished Report: Foundations and Medical Education 1909–1928." *Bulletin of the History of Medicine* 54 (1980): 475–96.

Gastel, B., and D. Rogers, eds. *Clinical Education and the Doctor of Tomorrow*. New York: The New York Academy of Medicine, 1989.

Gevitz, N. *The D.O.'s: Osteopathic Medicine in America*. Baltimore: Johns Hopkins University Press, 1982.

Hadley, J., ed. *Medical Education Financing*. New York: Prodist, 1980.

Harvey, A. *Science at the Bedside: Clinical Research in American Medicine 1905–1954*. Baltimore: Johns Hopkins University Press, 1981.

Hubbard, J. *Measuring Medical Education, 2nd edn*. Philadelphia: Lea Febiger, 1978.

Hudson, R. "Abraham Flexner in Perspective: American Medical Education 1865–1910." *Bulletin of the History of Medicine* 46 (1972): 545–61.

Hunt, A., and L. Weeks, eds. *Medical Education Since 1960: Marching to a Different Drummer*. East Lansing, Michigan: Michigan State Foundation, 1979.

Jarcho, S. "Medical Education in the United States, 1910–1956." *Journal of the Mt. Sinai Hospital* 26 (1959): 339–85.

Jolin, L. et al. "U.S. Medical School Finances." *JAMA* 266 (1991): 985–90.

Jonas, H., S. Etzel, and B. Barzansky. "Educational Programs in U.S. Medical Schools." *JAMA* 266 (1991): 913–923.

Jonas, S., ed. *Health Care Delivery in the United States, 3rd edn*. New York: Springer Publishing Company, 1986.

Kantrowitz, M. et al. *Innovative Tracks in Established Health Science Institutions: Strategies for Relevant Change*. Geneva: World Health Organization, 1987.

Kendall, P., and G. Reader. "Innovations in Medical Education in the 1950s Contrasted with Those of the 1970s and 1980s." *Journal of Health and Social Behavior* 29 (1988): 279–93.

Kett, J. *The Formation of the American Medical Profession: The Role of Institutions, 1780–1860*. New Haven: Yale University Press, 1968.

Kaufman, A., ed. *Implementing Problem-Based Medical Education*. New York: Springer Publishing Company, 1985.

Kaufman, M. *American Medical Education: The Formative Years, 1765–1910*. Westport, Connecticut: Greenwood Press, 1976.

Lee, P. *Medical Schools and the Changing Times*. Evanston, Illinois: Association of American Medical Colleges, 1962.

Lippard, V., and E. Purcell, eds. *The Changing Medical Curriculum*. New York: Josiah Macy Jr. Foundation, 1972.

Ludmerer, K. *Learning to Heal: The Development of American Medical Education.* New York: Basic Books, 1985.

Morantz-Sanchez, R. *Sympathy and Science: Women Physicians in American Medicine.* New York: Oxford University Press, 1985.

Muller, S. (Chairman). "Physicians for the Twenty-First Century: Report of the Project Panel on the General Professional Education of the Physician and College Preparation for Medicine." *Journal of Medical Education* 59, Part 2 (November 1984).

Perkoff. G. "Teaching Clinical Medicine in the Ambulatory Care Setting: An Idea Whose Time May Finally Have Come." *New England Journal of Medicine* 314 (1986): 27–31.

Report of the Graduate Medical Education National Advisory Committee (GMENAC), vols. 1–7 USDHHS Publication Nos. (HRA) 81–651 to 81–657. Washington, D.C.: USDHHS, 1980.

Rosenberg, C. *The Care of Strangers: The Rise of America's Hospital System.* New York: Basic Books, 1987.

Rothstein, W. *American Physicians in the Nineteenth Century: From Sects to Science.* Baltimore: Johns Hopkins University Press, 1972.

Rothstein, W. *American Medical Schools and the Practice of Medicine.* New York: Oxford University Press, 1987.

Shryock, R. *Medical Licensing in America, 1650–1965.* Baltimore: Johns Hopkins University Press. 1967.

Shryock, R. "The Influence of the Johns Hopkins University on American Medical Education." *Journal of Medical Education* 31 (1956): 226–35.

Scofield, J. *New and Expanded Medical Schools, Mid-Century to the 1980s.* San Francisco: Jossey Bass, 1984.

Smiley, D. "History of the Association of American Medical Colleges, 1896–1956. *Journal of Medical Education* 32 (1957): 512–25.

Starr, P. *The Social Transformation of American Medicine.* New York: Basic Books, 1982.

Stevens, R. *American Medicine and the Public Interest.* New Haven: Yale University Press, 1971.

Stevens, R. *In Sickness and in Wealth.* New York: Basic Books, 1989.

Waite, F. "Advent of the Graded Curriculum in American Medical Colleges." *Journal of the Association of American Medical Colleges* 25 (1950): 315–22.

Walsh, M. *Doctors Wanted: No Women Need Apply.* New Haven: Yale University Press, 1977.

Weiskotten, H. et al. *Medical Education in the United States, 1934–1939.* Chicago: American Medical Association, 1940.

Index

About the Contributors

ODIN W. ANDERSON is Professor of Sociology, University of Wisconsin-Madison. He is the author of several books including *Health Services in the United States* (1985) and *International Comparisons of Health Services* (1986).

EDWARD C. ATWATER is Associate Professor of Medicine and the History of Medicine, University of Rochester School of Medicine and Dentistry. He has published widely on the history of clinical medical education in America.

DEWITT C. BALDWIN, Jr. has served as Director, Division of Medical Education Research and Information, American Medical Association. He is senior editor of *Interdisciplinary Health Care Teams in Teaching* (1980) and *Interdisciplinary Health Team Training* (1982).

BARBARA BARZANSKY is Assistant Director of Undergraduate Medical Education, American Medical Association. She is co-author of *Innovation Processes in Medical Education* (1988).

NORMAN GEVITZ is Assistant Professor of the History of Medicine and Medical Education, University of Illinois College of Medicine. He is the author of *The D.O.'s: Osteopathic Medicine in America* (1982) and editor of *Other Healers: Unorthodox Medicine in America* (1988).

ROBERT P. HUDSON is Professor and Chairman, Department of History and Philosophy of Medicine, University of Kansas Medical Center. He is the author of *Disease and Its Control: The Shaping of Modern Thought* (1983).

DAVID A. KINDIG is Professor of Health Administration, Department of Preventive Medicine, University of Wisconsin. He has published widely in the area of medical manpower.

HORMOZ MOVASSAGHI is Assistant Professor of International Business, Ithaca College. Among his research interests are issues relating to the supply and distribution of physicians in the United States.

JANET D. PERLOFF is Associate Professor of Social Policy and Health Policy, School of Social Welfare and School of Public Health, State University of New York at Albany. She is senior author of *Medicaid and Pediatric Primary Care* (1987).

TODD L. SAVITT is Professor of the History of Medicine, Department of Medical Humanities, East Carolina University School of Medicine. He is the author of *Medicine and Slavery: The Diseases and Health Care of Blacks in Antebellum Virginia* (1978) and is senior editor of *Disease and Distinctiveness in the American South* (1988).

MARY ROTH WALSH is Professor of Psychology, University of Lowell. She is author of *Doctors Wanted: No Women Need Apply: Sexual Barriers in the Medical Profession* (1977) and editor of *The Psychology of Women: Ongoing Debates* (1987).